<u>sodium/potassium</u>
diet attracts male sperm
{bacon, beef, salmon, salty food}

<u>calcium</u>
diet attracts girl sperm
white meat, milk
dairy products

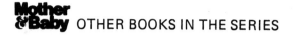

Mother & Baby OTHER BOOKS IN THE SERIES

QUESTIONS AND ANSWERS ON INFERTILITY

Dr. Alexander Gunn

ILLUSTRATED PUBLICATIONS
COMPANY LIMITED

© Illustrated Publications
Argus Books Ltd,
14 St James Road
Watford Herts

First published 1981

ISBN 0 85242 716 6

An Illustrated Publications book produced
by Argus Books Ltd, Watford, on behalf of
The Illustrated Publications Co Ltd,
12–18 Paul St, London, EC2A 4JS

Printed in Great Britain by
Thomson Litho Ltd, East Kilbride, Scotland

Contents

Introduction

Brought up to expect instant pregnancy as a result of 'unprotected' intercourse, many women are first of all surprised if this doesn't happen, then begin to worry as the months pass. Ultimately, after three, six, nine or more periods, it seems as if nature has let them down— 'am I doing something wrong?', 'should I see my doctor?', 'is there anything wrong with me—or my husband?'

The following letters and replies show clearly that a new problem is emerging for some young couples, not the old one of unwanted babies, but the new one of unwanted infertility.

CHAPTER I
The Range of Problems

Practical advice

Q.   I am 19 years old and have been married for one year. We have been trying for a baby for seven months. We are getting quite anxious to start a family while we are still young. Have you any suggestions? My periods are regular.
Mrs. K.C., Lancs.

A.   The normal fertile period for a woman is between 10 and 20 days after the first day of her last period, and if intercourse takes place regularly throughout this period of the menstrual calendar, the likelihood of conceiving is enhanced. If, however, after a period of a further six to nine months of consistently trying to start a family you do not have any success, it is time for you to consult your family doctor. He will then initiate all the appropriate tests on you and your husband to determine your fertility.

Reassurance

Q.   Could I be infertile? We've been married for over a year now, and most of my friends seem to have

started having babies very soon after they were married. I've never used any contraceptives and have begun to imagine there must be something wrong. Is there any way in which a couple should make love in order to get pregnant? When should I start to think of having investigations done?
Mrs. W.M., Notts.

A.   It is not at all uncommon for it to take longer than a year to conceive. Whilst one hears of many cases where conception occurs very rapidly, there are many many couples who are absolutely and perfectly normal who nevertheless have to wait very much longer before they conceive. You can't increase your chances of conception by making love in any special way. In fact, it is possible to conceive when seminal fluid is deposited only on the outside of the vagina and not necessarily high up inside as is more normal. You need not at this time even entertain thoughts of infertility. Most gynaecologists and doctors would advise a young couple that at least 18 months to two years should elapse before there is any necessity for any investigation of either partner. The most fertile period for a woman is from the 10th day after the onset of menstruation to the 20th, so concentrate on having intercourse during that part of the month, and it is possible that your efforts may be more successful.

Desperation

Q.   I am getting desperate. Every month I burst into tears with disappointment when my period starts—I do so want a family. I've been married for two years (I am 24) and there must be something wrong with me, or my husband, for we have been trying for a baby all the time. I'm becoming impossible to live with, and so bad tempered. The doctor is going to send me for some tests, but I am sure they will prove me to be infertile.
Mrs. B.M., Middlesex.

A.   Whilst there are many people who seem to

conceive almost instantly, there are many others for whom it takes longer. The fact that you are only 24 and have been married only for two years, means that since there is only one opportunity each month for conception to occur, you have really only had some two dozen or so opportunities so far, when in fact, out of your whole reproductive life, you have at least another 250 to go! So, at this stage in your life, you should not consider yourself infertile, nor should you assume that there is anything wrong with either you or your husband. I can well understand your worry and anxiety, but within the next few months when the tests are started you will begin to feel much more reassured.

Finding out

Q. What information can I get—and where can I get it from—that will help me to become pregnant? My husband and I are in our mid-twenties and we are beginning to think we might have a fertility problem—having tried for a baby for the last eight months or so now. Is there anything I could do—before getting involved with specialists? How could I find out if I am ovulating regularly for example?
Mrs. C.C., Midlands.

A. Your general practitioner or your local Family Planning Clinic would refer you to an infertility clinic if they felt it was necessary. However, you need not assume at this stage in your life that you are infertile, for with most young healthy couples, it really is only a matter of time before they do conceive.

One of the first things that you could do would be to keep a body temperature chart in order to plot your time of ovulation. For most women this is in the middle of the cycle, usually between the 10th and 14th day after the start of your previous period. The instructions that come with the charts are quite simple to follow and the completed charts also act as a most helpful guide to your medical advisers when you eventually are seen at the clinic. Your family doctor can give you copies of the chart and explain the way in which it should be completed.

Temperatures

Q. How do I keep an ovulation record? What sort of thermometer do I need, and how long does the record have to be kept?
Mrs. B.J., Norfolk.

A. You should buy an ordinary clinical thermometer from a chemist's shop and take your temperature—either in your mouth, or in your armpit—at the same time each morning, preferably on waking and prior to having any hot drinks, and writing down the precise temperature. If this is done regularly over a period of three months or so, (at the same time recording the days when menstruation takes place), you will see that some time between the 10th and the 14th day after the onset of menstruation, the body temperature drops by a point or two, and then rises again a day or two later. Provided there has been no infection to cause a rise in body temperature during that time, you will be able very clearly to predict the time at which an egg cell is released by your ovaries (ovulation), since this happens at the time of the alteration of temperature. In that way you will also be able to predict your most fertile period, for it is a few days either side of this change in body temperature (lasting for at least a week after the rise). If intercourse is frequent at this time, your chances of becoming pregnant are increased.

Various charts on which to record these temperatures are available from Family Planning Clinics and from your general practitioner, as well as explanatory booklets which may well also be helpful to you.

Timing

Q. When is the exact time that an egg cell is produced each month? Is it when the temperature rises, or when it falls? After an egg cell has been produced, how long can it remain capable of being fertilised?
Mrs. S.U., Devon.

A.   It is very difficult to be precise about the **exact** time of ovulation and its relation to a temperature change— I think it would probably take an experiment where women are cut open each month in order to determine what is happening, which is obviously totally impractical! However, to be more serious, it is fair to say that during the 48 hours of the temperature change (i.e., the drop and subsequent rise) from normal, an egg cell becomes available for fertilisation. How long it remains available is not certain, but from the evidence that some women conceive even as late as the day before an expected period, the egg cell's active existence must vary a lot—the average is, however, probably a week.

Operations

Q.   I am 22 and my husband is 27, and we have been trying to start a baby for the past nine months without success. A year ago I came off the pill, having been on it for two and a half years, and since then I appear to be ovulating normally.
The problem is that my periods have become progressively more painful and are accompanied by a sticky brown discharge just before and during the bleeding which usually lasts about five days. During the rest of my cycle I do not get any discharge. My GP suspects that I have an infection in my uterus and fallopian tubes and put me on a 10 day course of Erythromycin. He told me that if it did not clear up I would have to have a D & C.
I am very worried that my tubes might have got blocked up with this infection. Can you tell me if this is likely to happen? Also what does a D & C operation do? Does it improve fertility?
Mrs. H.C., London.

A.   The development of a brown discharge before your period, with no discharge at all during any other time, is not necessarily a sign of an infection. One would have expected, if there were an infection in the fallopian tubes or uterus, that the discharge would continue throughout the month and it may well be that your doctor is treating you with the antibiotic Erythromycin 'just in case', rather than with any certainty that an infection is present. There is no reason, therefore, for you to suspect a tubal blockage.

The dilation and curettage (D & C) operation is sometimes a very helpful diagnostic procedure, for it tends to open the cervix and, by scraping the lining of the uterus, leaves it in a healthier state to build up before implantation—thus it acts as an encouragement to conception as well as ascertaining that all is actually well inside.

Recovery

Q. Is there much bleeding after a D & C, and how long after it has been done do we have to wait before we can start trying for a baby again?
Mrs. B.G., Suffolk.

A. You will find that you have some small degree of vaginal loss for two or three days after this operation, very similar to a period, and as soon as this stops, it will be perfectly reasonable for you to resume sexual activity.

Infertility tests

Q. We are to have tests done at my hospital for infertility. My doctor explained briefly what they are going to do, but I thought perhaps you could give me more information, as at the moment I am getting quite nervous about it all.
Mrs. E.P., Exeter.

A. The usual tests for infertility are firstly analysis of your husband's semen after he has produced samples by masturbation, and secondly the recommendation that you keep a regular temperature chart in order to check whether you are ovulating. After that you will have various blood tests to determine your hormone levels, and, when these results are all available, you will have an internal examination to check on the health of your pelvic organs—the cervix and ovaries for example. Later, you may have to go to hospital for the day for an investigation as to whether your uterine tubes are clear and open. This is done by means of an X-ray of the genital passages which is taken during what is known as the insufflation test. This is where gas is blown gently into the uterine cavity and its presence is followed by serial X-rays to indicate whether the uterine tubes that lead to the ovary, are open, on either side. At the same time, under a general anaesthetic, a uterine scraping is done which is called a curettage, in order to detect whether the normal cells which line the uterus are in an appropriate phase according to the hormones controlling your monthly cycle.

Ovarian cysts

Q. I have been told that I might have an ovarian cyst and, if so, that it may be responsible for my failure to conceive and the pain I have been getting at period times. The hospital is admitting me for a 'laparoscopy' to find out. Could you tell me precisely what this entails, what are the symptoms of ovarian cysts and how are they dealt with? Will my fertility be affected afterwards? Mrs. R.M., Newcastle.

A. Basically this procedure involves a small incision being made in the abdominal wall, usually under a local, but sometimes under a general anaesthetic. The incision is not more than one inch wide and occasionally this can be done in the vaginal wall. A small flexible instrument about the thickness of a large fountain pen, is inserted through the incision, enabling the surgeon to carry out a full visual inspection of the internal pelvic organs, the state of the uterus, its tubes and the ovaries on both sides. Since, in your case, there has been a suggestion that an ovarian cyst might be present, this is a particularly good form of investigation, for cysts on the ovaries bulge like blisters from the ovarian surface and if it is a small one it is sometimes possible, with the same instrument, to electrically cauterise the cyst and therefore virtually remove it. On the other hand, if it is a larger one, and they do sometimes grow to the size of walnuts or even as big as small apples, it would then be necessary to perform an operation to remove the cyst. Ovarian cysts cause a variety of problems; obviously the larger ones can cause a great deal of difficulty, sometimes even twisting on themselves and becoming trapped, which means an acute abdominal emergency rather like an appendicitis. The smaller ones are troublesome however, in that they cause pain on deep penetration at intercourse, sometimes menstrual irregularity and quite frequently a degree of acute, deep-seated pain at the time of a period. This is because the tissue within the ovarian cyst is following the same pattern as the uterine lining and when the inside of the uterus bleeds, then the inside of the cyst bleeds as well, and this inevitably causes pain as well as a progressive increase in size of the ovarian cyst.

I am sure that the investigation will be very helpful in diagnosing any abnormality. I am sure, too, that once the cause has been dealt with, you will be in excellent health, for the removal of an ovarian cyst would undoubtedly improve your future fertility.

Long-term effects

Q. My daughter, who is only 12, had peritonitis last year after her appendix burst. She was desperately ill, and the surgeons said she nearly lost her life. She is fully recovered now, but I cannot help wondering whether her internal organs may have been permanently damaged. Will she be infertile when she grows up because of what she has been through? I know the ovaries are near the appendix and I cannot help worrying about any possible long-term effects.
Mrs. D.S., Sussex.

A. Your daughter may well not have suffered any damage to her ovaries as a result of her experience. Obviously some degree of scar tissue would have developed inside the lower part of her pelvis as a result of the peritonitis, but as she is only just about to enter puberty, the growth and development of her uterus and uterine tubes, as well as her ovaries, may not necessarily be in any way impaired as a result of this. She may, however start her periods a little later than others.

As I am sure you will appreciate, acute appendicitis is a very common disease and if every young girl, as a result, had her fertility seriously impaired, then infertility would be very much more common than it is.

Reduced fertility?

Q. Last year I had a severe appendicitis and an abscess formed. When I was operated on they had to remove my fallopian tube on that side as well. Does this mean I only have half the chance of becoming pregnant compared to anyone who has both tubes? How much has this reduced my fertility?
Mrs. C.M., Cheshire.

A. This operation inevitably diminishes the chances of the egg cells that your ovaries produce each month becoming fertilised. Nevertheless, it does not by any means reduce them by the apparently logical amount of 50 per cent. In fact, quite frequently, ovulation occurs and the egg cell appears in the remaining fallopian tube on alternate months or even in successive months, ready for fertilisation. If you wanted me to estimate the fertility reduction in percentage terms, it would only be reduced by about 25 per cent in comparison with normal.

Consolation

Q. I have just had to have an emergency operation, because I had an ectopic pregnancy and I think the tube had to be taken away. It was a bitter disappointment and now I know that my chances of becoming pregnant again are reduced. Could this problem recur if I did manage to conceive again? What are the chances of my having a baby eventually?
Mrs. N.P., Lincs.

A.   You did not say whether one of the ovaries had to be removed as well, and I would assume, therefore, that both ovaries are intact, although there is only one uterine tube present.

Your chances of becoming pregnant again are, in fact, statistically only partially reduced by comparison to what they would be if you had two fallopian tubes. A reduction of one in four, or 25 per cent would be a realistic estimate of your operation's effect on your fertility. Ovulation still occurs just as regularly and in alternate months at least an ovum is released by the ovary into the remaining fallopian tube adjacent to it—therefore there is no reason whatsoever why you should not become pregnant in due course.

Despite this setback, you have demonstrated the fertility of both you and your husband. There is no reason to assume that an ectopic pregnancy will occur again, so you have every confidence that next time you conceive, things will proceed normally.

Fibroids

Q.   I am 33, and after trying to become pregnant for the last three years I eventually saw a specialist. He has found that I have a fibroid in the uterus and thinks this might be responsible for my failure to conceive. He has suggested an operation to remove it. A friend of mine with fibroids, however, has had two children and she has never had any problems. Why is this? Could you tell me precisely what fibroids are, why they affect fertility and what the operation entails?
Mrs. W. T., Midlands.

A.   Fibroids are small non-malignant fibrous over-growths of the uterine muscle, occurring quite commonly. They can, however, cause problems with conception, the progress of a pregnancy, and in the early post-natal period. Since they occupy a certain amount of space in the uterine wall, they reduce the size of the uterine cavity, and so may provoke a miscarriage, because they prevent the development and growth of the foetus in its early weeks.

For that reason, it is usually advised that any large fibroid is removed prior to conception. The only dilemma about this advice is that it is necessary to make a small incision in the wall of the uterus in order to remove the fibroid. This incision can be a natural weakness, for a few months after the operation, and it is desirable, therefore, to leave at least a three to six months gap after the fibroid's removal before becoming pregnant, for only by then will the incision have completely healed.

The operation involves a small incision across the lower part of the abdomen (somewhat similar to that left after a Caesarean operation) and then by a simple cut down the surface of the uterus, over the fibroid, the fibroid is easily removed. The two incisions are then carefully and firmly stitched up. It is usual to be in hospital for seven days or less, and there is perhaps another week or 10 days or so after discharge from hospital before you can resume all your normal activities, for it is natural after this type of operation to feel tired, the scar is tender, and you must be careful about heavy lifting and hard physical work.

Quite frequently, however, due to the hormonal influences in pregnancy, a small fibroid collapses and shrinks on its own. For that reason, therefore, women with relatively small fibroids are frequently advised to ignore them in the hope that this spares them the necessity of an operation.

Husband's fertility

Q. After trying for a family for over a year without success, we have just been given the shattering news that my husband is sub-fertile.
He is at the moment waiting to see a consultant at our local hospital, but we feel at a loss to understand why this has happened to him. Is there any treatment at the moment which can improve a man's fertility? We feel that this news is the end of the world for us.
Mrs. M.J., Hants.

A. There are many levels of fertility in men, from those

19

who produce perfectly normal sperm counts to those who have very, very low sperm counts indeed. Your husband has been told that he is sub-fertile, not infertile, and one must presume that he is producing some sperm, at least on some occasions. This is reassuring because it only takes one sperm for a conception to occur.

The number of sperms which a man produces can be increased by the use of male sex hormones, and certain new drugs have recently become available. Although their success is not guaranteed, in general they do produce an improvement in the sperm count when they are taken over a considerable period of time, and I am sure that when your husband sees the consultant, these new kinds of treatments will be discussed.

A low sperm count

Q.   My husband has a low sperm count, (about 600), and our doctor tells us we have very little chance of having children, but he has given my husband a course of Proviron tablets. As yet they don't seem to have done any good. We have been married for eight years. For the last two, we have been hoping for a family. I have started taking my temperature every morning to see if I can find the best time for intercourse. Is there anything else we could try, or any other tablets my husband could try?
Mrs. F.T., Scotland.

A.   The fact that your husband had a sperm count of 600 on one occasion is hopeful, for although this is on the low side, it does demonstrate the possibility of you becoming pregnant by normal means. Proviron is helpful since it was designed to improve the sperm count, and I would certainly not give up hope yet. This is a new preparation, and at present it is one of the best available. I would recommend that you continue taking your temperature regularly in order to work out your most fertile period. It would be helpful, however, for both you and your husband to be referred by your doctor to an infertility clinic. The simple testing of one sperm sample, is not, I feel, the answer to a couple's problems where conception is delayed. There are other forms of treatment and assessment, and the specialists at a clinic are best able to help you and your husband in this matter.

Too low?

Q. I have just had the results of my husband's sperm count. He has about a '20 per cent active' count. Following this, my husband was told to wear cotton underwear, have no hot baths and to wear looser clothing. Does this really help? Is his sperm count too low for me to become pregnant?
Mrs. M.B., Wilts.

A. Your husband's sperm count is, in fact, relatively reassuring, for 100 per cent activity is very rarely seen, and the average is between 40 and 60 per cent. As sperm activity can be influenced by the frequency of ejaculation, or the time interval between the production of the sample and its examination in the laboratory, a 20 per cent count would be considered to be only a little on the low side, and certainly not one that would be regarded as infertile.
It is quite true that if the scrotum is not kept too warm and in too close a position to the body, the sperm count tends to rise, but in fact these factors have only a very small effect on fertility. In your husband's case, bearing in mind that it requires only one spermatozoa of the 50 million or so produced with each ejaculation, to achieve fertilisation, there is no reason whatsoever why you should not become pregnant at any time.

Obsessed

Q. Some time ago when I wrote to you, you really gave me hope and confidence regarding my chances of getting pregnant. This was my attitude when I attended the sub-fertility clinic for a series of tests to be started and I felt quite excited that, at last, something was being done. I was kept waiting for over an hour, then told to undress and wait to be called. Whilst waiting I could hear a lot of shouting and arguing and my name was mentioned several times. Eventually I was called in to see the doctor only to be told that I had been referred to the wrong clinic and wrong doctor, and that, at 22 days after my last period, it was the wrong time of the month for the test they wanted to do to be carried out. The doctor very grudgingly carried out the test none too gently, whilst treating me like some kind of imbecile and warned me that the result would be inaccurate. I felt very humiliated, not to mention disappointed, and although I have been given another appointment for another test I don't want to go. I really am fed up with the treatment I've received at this clinic, and it has destroyed all the confidence your advice instilled in me and made me very unhappy. In fact, I think it has set me back into the state I was in before. My husband feels exactly the same as I do, whereas before he at least remained fairly optimistic.

I feel I'm becoming obsessed with the problem once more. There doesn't seem to be any purpose in life without children, and at times I feel I can't stand this intolerable situation any longer. Also, this month, my period was overdue by a week and whilst one part of me was hoping I could be pregnant, the other part of me knew it was probably due to the upset I had at the hospital. I don't think I'm any nearer to getting pregnant now than I was three years ago. Can you suggest anything we can do, or a specialist we could see? We would be prepared to pay for treatment if it would give us a baby. I hope you can offer me some advice as I'm feeling really down and miserable.

Mrs. T.W., Worcs.

A. I do feel that many doctors fail to recognise how sensitive and upset women can be who are patients at a sub-fertility clinic, and certainly I can appreciate how your confidence has taken a severe jolt as a result of what you went through. I would still advise you to persist, for I have little doubt that in the end, when you do conceive and ultimately carry a pregnancy through to term, all the unpleasantness that you are having to put up with at the moment will be forgotten.

Your feelings are shared by a very large number of

women indeed, all of whom, secretly more often than not, are feeling the same as you because they are childless. As you are already on the way to having access to the necessary investigations for sub-fertility, you should not consider getting involved with expensive private specialists yet (if indeed you ever have to). Bear with it all for just a little longer until the results of your tests are available. Once these are to hand you could then ask your family doctor to arrange one private appointment for you and your husband with the senior specialist, so that you could have a full and frank discussion, as well as an interpretation of all the scientific findings (although I would warn you that this might well cost around £30 to £35 or so).

CHAPTER II

Menstrual Irregularity after the Pill

Pill worries

Q.   I feel reluctant to visit my own doctor about this matter as I fear he may consider my anxiety premature, but having read about the infertility that can be caused by long-term taking of the pill, I am beginning to wonder if my fertility may have been affected.

I have been on the pill for almost nine years without more than the occasional break and recently decided to try to have a baby. My periods started spontaneously, but have been slightly irregular, 30 days, 28 days and 32 days. We have tried for two months to have a baby and I suppose we may have missed ovulation, (if indeed that is taking place). We have intercourse at least three to four times a week.

How likely is it that I could be menstruating without ovulating? How frequently is a woman made infertile after taking the pill for a long period? My periods were regular, about every 24/25 days before I went on the pill, and I had no trouble with them at all. How soon could I be checked to make sure that I am not infertile? I was horrified to see that some doctors will not refer a young couple to a sub-fertility clinic until two years of attempts to have a baby have proved fruitless. I am $28\frac{1}{2}$ years old and quite healthy, as is my husband. There is no history of infertility on either side of the family and the relatives on my side seem to have conceived (even when taking what should have been reasonably adequate precautions) with ease.

Mrs. F.T., Surrey.

A.   The Royal College of General Practitioners' survey of some 50,000 pregnancies occurring over eight years demonstrated that infertility cannot be due to the pill. Because the oral contraceptive is such an effective form of fertility control, it can carry women through the most fertile period of their lives, so that when they do want to conceive, they may then be less fertile than they were several years before. This is a consequence of time and not of the medication, and in your case, as you are still young, I would suggest that it will not be very long before you do conceive.

As to whether you might be menstruating without ovulating, the simple answer to this is to keep a temperature chart. If you did this for three months or so, you would most likely see that ovulation was occurring. If after a further six months you have still not conceived, then you should ask your family doctor to refer you to a specialist. You can also ask for such help at a Family Planning Clinic (whose address is in the local telephone book) who are developing this side of their work. I am sure you will realise that having really only had two chances to become pregnant—as you have only been trying to conceive for the last two months—you may have to wait a little longer.

Too long?

Q.   I have been married for seven years, and for the first five years of my married life I was on the pill. I stopped taking the pill over two years ago, but despite having taken no contraceptive precautions since, no pregnancy has resulted.

My periods have always been regular from the age of 10 and returned 28 days from the last pill-induced period. During the last year I have kept regular temperature charts which indicate the normal fall and rise in temperature during the month. My only previous gynaecological history is an operation for a cervical erosion six years ago. This had caused no symptoms but was discovered in a routine examination.

I have had an initial consultation with a consultant gynaecologist, and a physical examination revealed no apparent abnormalities except that the erosion had returned. The specialist suggested a D & C to be performed in the third week of the menstrual cycle and the erosion to be cauterised at the same time. Incidentally, all my blood tests and my husband's sperm count have proved to be normal. My husband and I are both aged 30 and are in good health. My main concerns are as follows:—

    a) Has taking the pill for as long as five years jeopardised my chances of having a baby?

    b) Would it be dangerous for me to conceive a child with an existing cervical erosion?

    c) How could a D & C operation help in alleviating the infertility problem?

    d) The first period I had subsequent to my last operation for the cervical erosion was extremely heavy and prolonged. Is this likely to happen again or be even worse in view of the fact that it is suggested that the operation take place in the third week of the menstrual cycle?

Mrs. R.S., Notts.

A.   The oral contraceptive does not impair subsequent fertility in a woman after she has finished taking it. One thing, however, that must be recognised is that you have been carried through what may be the most fertile years of your life completely protected from the possibility of conception because of the pill.

However, you still have many reproductive years left, and you have shown that you ovulate regularly. The fact that all your blood tests and your husband's sperm count have also proved to be normal, is most reassuring and I am quite certain, therefore, that you will conceive in due course.

In answer to your specific queries, taking the pill has certainly not jeopardised your chances of having a baby in the long term, and there is no danger whatsoever in your conceiving when a minor degree of cervical erosion is still present (although once the erosion is corrected by cautery, after you have had the D & C operation, your chances of conceiving will be enhanced).

Thirdly, the dilation of the cervix (which is an essential part of this operation) also improves the chances of conception, but the curettage is used to obtain cells from the lining of the uterus at a particular point in the menstrual calendar. This is very helpful to see whether, in fact, what is called the 'proliferative' stage of the uterine lining's development (which normally occurs in the third week of a menstrual cycle) is developing appropriately. Should this not be the case, a hormonal supplement would be prescribed. Finally, it is likely that you will have a heavier menstrual period than usual immediately after the D & C and quite probably this will continue until your period starts.

Erosions

Q. I am 26, and my husband is coming up to 30. We have been married for two years. We would very much like to start a family, and I stopped taking the pill three months ago. So far, nothing has happened, despite making love at what I understood to be the most likely time (just before the half-way point between periods). I started taking the pill six years ago, after becoming pregnant very easily. At the time, I had an abortion and I wonder if this is anything to do with not becoming pregnant when actually trying, as ironically, I was more or less a virgin the first time.

I understand that there is a method of pinpointing the time of ovulation by taking one's temperature. Since stopping the pill, my periods have become irregular, making it difficult to assess the 'half-way mark'. Would you kindly answer the following questions:—
1) How often should the temperature be taken, so as not to miss the 'rise and fall'?
2) How long is the interval between the temperature rising and falling, and how much does it fluctuate?
3) How long is the fertile period? I have heard vary-

ing opinions—from 12 hours per month to about five days?

4) How long do the sperms remain active in the woman's body after intercourse?

5) While attending check-ups some time after my abortion regarding a vaginal discharge, I was told there was a slight erosion of the cervix. I used various pessaries and pills, to no avail. Would this hinder conception in any way?

Mrs. R.L., Yorks.

A.   Having stopped taking the pill only three months ago, you have had little more than three opportunities to become pregnant, and in view of the fact that many people, particularly once they are out of their teens, sometimes take 18 months to two years to become pregnant, you need not at this stage become too anxious. Your abortion six years ago is most unlikely to have anything to do with your not having become pregnant yet. In fact, it demonstrates that you are fertile, which is reassuring.

The method of pinpointing the time of ovulation is really fairly simple, and it requires only a standard clinical thermometer from any chemist. Use it every day, and preferably at the same time each day, to accurately record the body's temperature. The temperature should be taken in the same way, perhaps on waking, in your mouth before you have any cups of tea or breakfast, and you then record it with the date throughout each month. If you do this for about three months, you will find that a regular pattern emerges. The body's temperature is usually 98.4 (36.7) degrees, but some time between the 10th and 14th day after the start of a period, the temperature drops perhaps to 97.5 (36.2) degrees or so, and then rises on the following day to 98.9 (36.9) degrees. This shows that ovulation has occurred.

The fertile period can last as long as a week or 10 days, and sperm can remain active in your body after intercourse for two to three days, or even longer.

Finally, if you are still suffering from the vaginal discharge, ask your family doctor for a check on this, such as a cervical smear and a swab, and if the minor erosion of the cervix is still present, he will refer you to a gynaecologist for treatment. It does not necessarily hinder conception, but it would be better if this were cleared up prior to the pregnancy, as a healthy genital tract certainly offers a better chance of conception than one with minor disorders.

A past abortion

Q. I am 28 and have been married for 12 months. We have been trying for a baby for that time with no success. I had a termination four years ago, when I was seven weeks pregnant. It was not my husband's pregnancy, and he knows nothing about it. There were no complications, and immediately afterwards I went on the pill. I took this for three years. When I stopped, my periods were very irregular and scanty. There was no pain or discomfort. I put this down to a delay in ovulation.

My doctor suggested taking my temperature for a month, but as I am a night nurse, this was neither very accurate nor convenient.

Recently my periods have gradually become regular in a 30-32 day cycle lasting four to five days. My loss is dark brown mixed with blood and this does worry me a little. I sometimes get breast discomfort and tenderness —also some increase in vaginal secretions a day or two before. Do you think it too early yet to return to my doctor for further more thorough investigations? My cycle was perfectly regular before I took the pill, being 28-29 days. Could my past termination, or the pill, have affected my fertility?

Mrs. A.B., Lancs.

A. Neither your previous gynaecological history, nor your use of the pill is likely to have impaired your fertility. Indeed your previous conception demonstrates your ability to become pregnant. The irregularity which you experienced with your menstrual cycle after taking the pill probably means that you did not have any opportunity to conceive during those particular cycles— for ovulation may not have taken place. It would seem that it is only recently, since your periods became regular, that you have had the opportunity to conceive and as a rough estimate, therefore, you have probably only had some six or seven chances.

I suggest you keep a regular temperature chart in order to detect ovulation, for at least three to four months, before asking your doctor for any other form of investigations. I can appreciate how concerned you are as each period arrives, but I am sure you will see that your chances of conceiving have been rather few, and the time to initiate investigations and any form of treatment should it prove necessary, will be in another six to nine months or so.

Pill reaction

Q. What does the pill do to a woman's body? Are the hormones harmful, and why do they stop the periods after a woman has been on it? How long do the periods stop for? I came off it three months ago and have not had a period yet, but we want a baby—should I have a pregnancy test? What worries me most is that I have two friends who took the pill and have now been told they are sterile.
Mrs. S.J., Midlands.

A. Taking an oral contraceptive is, in fact, adding extra hormones to a woman's body, and therefore her own production of these hormones diminishes slightly —once she stops taking the pill it is common for some time to elapse before her body resumes responsibility for control of the menstrual cycle. Suppression of menstruation after stopping the pill can occasionally go on for as long as one to two years, but in most cases normal periods return within three to six months.

As it is only some three months since you stopped taking the pill, it is early days for you as yet, and you may find that in another two or three months or so your menstrual cycle begins again. It is possible, of course, to ovulate without menstruation so a woman can be fertile even though she is not having a period, so it is quite sensible for you to have a pregnancy test from time to time just to check on this. With regard to your two friends who you tell me have been 'sterile' since they took the pill, I must stress that the pill does not have any suppressive effect on a woman's fertility once she stops taking it; (in fact, there is often the opposite effect with 'rebound' ovulation occurring leading to an enhancement of fertility rather than a reduction.) I would suggest, therefore, that there may well be some other reason for the infertility of your friends, and that the oral contraceptives are being unfairly and wrongly blamed.

The injection

Q.   We are trying for a baby now, but I was given a birth control injection which lasts for about three months, a year ago. The clinic told me I would be 'safeguarded' for three months only, after which I would have to go on to the pill if I wanted continued contraception. When I left the clinic to go home, I was bleeding heavily. Three months after the birth control injection I was still bleeding and I was put on the pill by the Family Planning Clinic. I came off the pill seven months after the birth control injection but I was still bleeding, then it stopped suddenly on its own. My periods are only just beginning to be normal now (approx. 28-30 day cycle, five to six days' bleeding).
My husband is 26, I am 24; we're both in good health but there's still no baby, despite nearly a year of trying. I went to my GP today to see if anything could be done, but he suggested it could be the birth control injection that is causing the delay in conception.
I was not warned about any side effects from this drug, and was told it would only last three months and not a whole year. How long will it be before I am likely to be able to conceive—will this injection continue to affect me?
Mrs. D.J., Scotland.

A.   You certainly seem to have suffered from the side-effects of the contraceptive injection and it is obvious that the hormones it contains have totally upset your system. Your fertility will not be impaired in the long term at all, but until your menstrual pattern settles down to normal, it's unlikely that you will conceive. You can, however, be confident that once these present side effects are over, your body will return to normal and you should have very little difficulty then in becoming pregnant.

Ask your doctor for a referral to a gynaecologist if your symptoms persist for very much longer, because occasionally further forms of treatment to make the hormonal system settle down can help in cases like yours. However, if the more normal cycle you mention persists, then I would hope that pregnancy would occur within the next six months.

Still no periods

Q. Earlier this year I came off the pill but I did not have a period as I would have expected. During the next couple of months I had three pregnancy tests, two negative followed by a positive result on the third occasion. I was delighted, but to my dismay, a month later I had what I can only describe as another period. I contacted my GP who advised rest and told me I had a threatened miscarriage. I took as much rest as possible, but the loss lasted for four days (I had no pain). I then had another pregnancy test which proved negative. I now find my next period is nearly a week overdue. As I have to wait for another week to a fortnight before I can return to my GP I would appreciate your opinion. I lost no clots or tissue or anything like that during my 'period'—is it possible my pregnancy is still progressing, or is this perhaps just a delayed period, or could it be a completely new pregnancy altogether? I am somewhat bewildered by now. Is there anything I can do to establish whether or not I am pregnant once and for all, because the uncertainty is driving me mad?
Mrs. H.G., London.

A. This is quite a common experience for women who have been taking the pill, and menstrual irregularity often continues for at least three to six months after stopping the pill. From what you tell me, I doubt whether you are pregnant at the moment, or indeed ever have been, unless you are having any other symptoms besides menstrual irregularity.

Ask your family doctor to refer you to a gynaecologist for an assessment, in case any other treatment might be necessary to regularise your periods and to assist your hormonal cycle back to normality. The treatment of menstrual suppression is nowadays quite sophisticated, and this might be helpful for you.

When to stop

Q. We are keen to have a baby and wonder if you could advise me which would be the best part of the cycle to stop taking the pill to give the maximum chance of conception?
Mrs. K.S., Lincs.

A. You should stop taking the pill at least two to three months before you hope to conceive, and the best time to stop is when you have reached the end of the pack as it is not possible to ensure that ovulation will occur in any cyclical or predictable pattern if you stop halfway through. A time interval of two to three months is necessary, because the pill's hormones often take that long to disappear from your body, and also your own hormones will probably take about the same amount of time to resume their activity and restart ovulation. Indeed, few women conceive in the first three months or so after stopping the pill.

Herbal help?

Q. I have not had a period for three months, although I have never before missed a period in my life. I was advised by my doctor to have a pregnancy test, which proved negative. He then gave me some hormone tablets to bring on menstruation—five days later I had a brown discharge but no bleeding. I have been taking my temperature for the last three months but have not ovulated.
Why have I suddenly ceased to menstruate, and what

is the cause of the hormonal imbalance? I have read that herbal remedies have been successful, but will I have to live with infertility and hormonal imbalance for the rest of my reproductive years? I am 37. Should I see a specialist?

A.   It certainly seems that your hormones are upset, and the treatment you have received apparently has not yet helped to bring your periods back to normal. I don't think that herbal remedies have a great deal to offer in your case. This may be just a temporary phase, and the best action is to do nothing and wait for the present hormonal imbalance to settle down.

Emotional upset, worry, change of life style and many other factors can be responsible for a woman's periods stopping temporarily. If your periods do not restart in the next three months, you should then seek referral to a gynaecologist.

However, there is no need to feel that this is the end of your reproductive life, for it is rare for the menopause to start as early as the late thirties.

Pregnant or not?

Q.   Is it possible to have periods and yet be pregnant? I have been trying for a baby for the best part of a year now by using the temperature method to detect the time of ovulation. However, at the time my period was due, I had slight spotting and lost nothing during the first night; this was followed by three or four days of light bleeding with no pain. The latter is unusual as I always suffer a great deal of pain at this time. The second month brought virtually the same, so I went to my GP for a pregnancy test, which proved negative. As the third month was approaching I naturally hoped there wouldn't be a period, no matter how slight, but much to my surprise it arrived late (as had the second one) but this time it was just like my usual periods (heavy and painful). At first I felt very distressed but then a friend told me she had had periods all through pregnancy. In the normal way I would have given up all hopes of being pregnant, but I have two 'symptoms'

which make me very confused. Firstly, I have noticed that glands around my nipples have appeared and seem to be increasing in size and number. The nipples also seem to have whitish patches on them and a yellowish liquid can easily be squeezed from them. Perhaps the most encouraging but confusing thing is that for about the last three weeks my abdomen has looked very pregnant! At first it was only noticeable at night, but now it is quite distended in the daytime too. I don't wish to see my GP again until I know whether it is possible to have periods and still be pregnant. I kept on recording my temperature chart during the last two months and the rise due to ovulation is not clear any more. I have no idea if or when I am ovulating—which will make it impossible to work out the right time to conceive. Does one ovulate during pregnancy?
Mrs. B.E., Scotland.

A.   When conception occurs a small part of the ovary and a small part of the developing placenta secrete hormones which signal to the brain that there is no necessity for menstruation to take place. If these chemical signals are not strong enough, menstruation can occur, either at the normal time or sometimes a little late and a woman can, therefore, miscarry. It is estimated that something like one third of all conceptions actually get swept away because of this hormonal deficiency, and of those remaining, a further 20 per cent are miscarried later (often between the eighth and 12th week) because the chemical signals, or hormones, are too weak. Where everything goes well, a woman has no further menstrual periods after conception, but there are cases where conception occurs, pregnancy continues and the periods apparently take place, but, more often than not, these periods are different from the normal ones. The usual difference is that they are delayed, very much shortened, rarely consist of the full, red menstrual flow, are not painful and usually consist mostly of brownish loss, lasting for not longer than a day and a half. Pregnancy tests depend on the detection of sufficient of the pregnancy hormones in the urine, and quite frequently a negative result can come about if there is not enough hormone present for the test to react. Nevertheless, as the pregnancy advances, the hormone levels inevitably increase and the tests become positive. In your case, I am afraid it is almost impossible to give a precise answer as to whether you may be pregnant or not. Certainly the symptoms of breast change may well be compatible with pregnancy, but as you do not indicate whether your periods are exactly normal or changed in any way, it is even more difficult to be precise. The increase in your waist size is not a symptom positively associated with pregnancy; more likely signs would be, morning nausea, frequency in passing urine or perhaps an increase in vaginal secretions.

The most sensible thing would be to ask your general practitioner to have the pregnancy test repeated. Your temperature chart would not be, in any case, as reliable a guide as a positive test, but its going haywire probably is a reflection of your hormonal irregularity.

Irregular periods

Q. Whenever doctors write about fertile periods they always seem to assume that a woman has regular menstruation. What about the woman with irregular periods—does she not have a fertile time, too? Also, can you please tell me if having intercourse too frequently reduces the chances of conceiving? When, if a woman has irregular periods, would be the best time in the cycle for intercourse?
Mrs. F.C., Berks.

A. You don't have to have regular periods before you can predict your most fertile time. If you keep an accurate daily temperature chart this will show you the most fertile period in your calendar. For example, whilst a woman may well have a period every 28 days or so, a temperature chart usually shows that the small dip and rise in the daily reading occurs at some time between the 10th and 14th day after her period started. However, even for the most regular woman, it is necessary to continue this form of charting for at least three months to see whether ovulation occurs each month at around the same time. If it does, then she can assume that this is her most fertile time. On the other hand, if a woman has very irregular periods, it is only by taking her daily temperature that she can find what relationship there is between ovulation and the ending of each period. She might find that whilst menstruation is irregular, ovulation is not, but still occurs around 10 to 14 days after the previous period.

In other words, a constant relationship can exist between the onset of menstruation and ovulation regardless of the time between periods.

Finally, concerning intercourse, it can't really occur so frequently as to inhibit fertility, and my own feelings are that no couple who are trying to conceive should become slaves to their temperature chart.

Changed pattern

Q.   Since my daughter was born two years ago, my periods have changed drastically and I wonder if this means my fertility has been reduced? I used to have a 28 day cycle—now it is nearly 36 days. Is this normal? We've been trying for another baby now for six months without success.
Mrs. P.A., Yorks.

A.   The changed pattern you describe is not at all uncommon after pregnancy. Provided your cycle is regular there is no need for concern about its length at all. Like all averages, the 'normal' cycle allows for deviations both below and above, often varying by as much as a week or more. Similarly, there is no reason to assume that your fertility is in any way impaired, but it must be recognised that whilst women usually find it fairly easy to conceive their first child, the conception of the second child may take a year to two years or so, despite regular menstruation.

Breast-feeding effect

Q.   I want another baby very soon. My son was born nine months ago and was fully breast-fed for six

months, but my periods have not yet returned. I still give him an evening breast-feed, and I have had two scanty periods, but when will my periods get back to normal? Am I ovulating at the moment?
Mrs. R.S., Lincs.

A.   Having entirely breast-fed your son for six months, your hormones are geared to breast milk production, rather than to egg cell production; menstruation will not occur while a woman is breast-feeding her baby completely. As you are still partially breast-feeding your son, this is still stimulating the lactating hormones, which is why you are not yet having regular periods. Once you have entirely stopped breast-feeding, your periods will return within one to two months and probably be as they were before your pregnancy. After three normal cycles, you can expect a very high likelihood of conception. Having already proved that both you and your husband are fertile, you should have no difficulty in conceiving in due course.

Hormonal upset

Q.   I am now 28 and married five years ago, but for the last two years, my periods have been chaotic. I have never been on the pill, and we have been trying to have a baby for 18 months but everything seems to be wrong with me. Not only are my periods irregular but my breasts hurt often for weeks on end and I get very tired, irritable and have even felt sick in the mornings. I I keep hoping it's a pregnancy starting, then my period comes. What is causing all this?
Mrs. D.T., Lancs.

A.   Your menstrual irregularity, the breast tenderness, the fatigue and the nausea, would suggest that you have some minor degree of hormonal abnormality. This is something that can be corrected, and in view of the fact that you have now been trying to conceive for the last 18 months, you should ask your family doctor to refer you to a gynaecologist. Your menstrual irregularity and minor hormonal disorder are by no means serious, but are probably playing a part in your failure to conceive.

The most likely treatment would be a hormone preparation, probably to be taken for a period of three to four months, in order to stabilise your menstruation. During that time you would be unlikely to conceive, but once the treatment was completed you could expect conception to occur with much greater ease than without treatment or investigation.

Hormonal excess

Q. I get very painful breasts—tender and swollen each month. Sometimes a little fluid comes from the nipples, but rarely have periods. I am 38 and having just got married would dearly love a baby—is it my hormones that are responsible for the fact that I do not menstruate regularly, and can anything be done about it?
Mrs. H.R., Hants.

A. I think you probably suffer from an excess of a hormone known as prolactin. This hormone can suppress menstruation and so obviously impairs fertility. The excess secretion of this hormone can be corrected by a type of fertility drug which suppresses prolactin, and which a gynaecologist can prescribe for you. It is by no means too late for you to have this form of treatment and whilst, naturally, it is a little more difficult for a woman of your age to conceive as promptly as if you were much younger, nevertheless, the right treatment will help you to do so.

Hormonal disorder

Q. Since the birth of my son a year ago we have not been too concerned about birth control. I had my first period, after a lot of spotting, when he was five months old and I tried one month on the pill and felt frightful—my neck ached constantly and my breasts throbbed. My period came four days before the course of pills was

finished, and I was permanently bursting into tears.
Since then—six months now—we have used no contraception and have now reached the stage where I am
trying to conceive. My periods are now going in six- or
seven-week cycles, but for the week or so beforehand,
I feel sick, my breasts feel full and I feel nauseous. I have
also started to leak milk from one of my breasts although
it had previously dried up. I get terrific period pain a
fortnight before—at around four weeks. I wonder if I am
ovulating—and is there something wrong with my
hormones?
Mrs. W.K., Sussex.

A.   Your menstrual cycle is apparently liable to bouts of
abnormality, shown by the irregular gaps between your
periods. It is also significant that you found the pill
unpleasant, and this tends to confirm a disorder in your
hormonal profile. Your premenstrual tension, nausea and
evidence of lactation in the breasts, as well as the period
pain, all fit in with a diagnosis of a prolactin hormone
excess. This is now becoming a much more widely
recognised condition, which is responsible for menstrual
irregularity, comparative infertility, painful periods, pre-
menstrual tension and breast milk secretion. There are
now various blood tests available to measure prolactin
hormone levels, and you should ask your doctor to refer
you to a specialist for this form of investigation. Treatment with a new substance known as Bromocryptine is
very effective, restoring a normal menstrual cycle,
ovulation and the possibility of successful conception.

Tablet worries

Q.   I am taking Duphaston (which I believe are
hormone tablets) to correct irregular bleeding. As we
are hoping for a baby I have been taking my temperature
in the morning, and it appears I am not ovulating—
hence the irregular bleeding. I have two worries. Firstly,
if I should ovulate and become pregnant whilst taking
the tablets would they in any way harm the baby?
Secondly, my temperature did drop markedly just
before I started taking the tablets so I might have
ovulated then and possibly have become pregnant. Will

the tablets have harmed me in any way—and how long should I go on keeping the chart, before I seek any other sort of help?
Mrs. C.R., Cumbria.

A.   If you conceive whilst taking Duphaston tablets, they would in no way harm the developing foetus, for they simply contain one of the female sex hormones, progestogen, which is in fact sometimes used to prevent a miscarriage and has no harmful effect on an early pregnancy.

It often takes between six and 18 months to conceive and whilst it is important to continue keeping a temperature chart for guidance, you will appreciate that this period of time has to elapse before any other form of intervention is considered necessary.

Duphaston does actually stimulate fertility and if, after some six months or so, you have still failed to conceive, you should ask your general practitioner to refer you to a gynaecologist for another form of hormonal supplementation.

Irregular

Q.   After my second son was born 17 months ago, my periods appeared to settle into a normal pattern, but then seven months after the birth they became increasingly irregular, their main feature being a tendency to brownish staining for two to four days before the period started properly. They also became less predictable and rather heavier. My doctor prescribed Dicynene to be taken when I estimated the spotting would start, to try to cut this out completely. Will this reduce my fertility in any way or damage the baby if I did conceive?
Mrs. F.J., Wales.

A.   Dicynene is not likely to prove harmful if you conceive. It is not a hormonal product, and although it acts in a rather complicated way to reduce the amount of menstrual loss, there is no evidence to suggest that it can be damaging to a pregnancy, or that it reduces fertility.

CHAPTER III

After a Miscarriage

Why miscarriages occur

Q.   Six months ago I had a miscarriage at seven weeks, and one month ago I had a second miscarriage at nine weeks. After the first, I was told by my GP to wait three months before trying again, which we did. When I conceived again the doctor was not sure if it was in the fourth or fifth month as I had had a very scanty period between those two months.
I have been given no tests to see if there is anything wrong with me to cause a miscarriage, and I am worried that when we try again I might miscarry once more. I know my miscarriages have happened in the early weeks of pregnancy, but I would still like to know if possible, before I conceive again, what has caused them.
Mrs. M.C., Northumbria.

A.   The reasons for a miscarriage are many and varied. In some cases it is due to a genetic accident which produces a foetal abnormality; in others it is due to an impairment in the health of the mother, and in many cases it is entirely inexplicable. In your case, however, your history would tend to suggest that your hormonal profile had not quite returned to normal after your first miscarriage before you conceived again. When there is some degree of hormonal insufficiency, the tendency to miscarry is increased. For that reason, therefore, I suggest that you wait at least three and possibly six months, before you try to conceive again in order to allow your body and its hormones to return to normal. Once your periods are regular and once you miss your first period with pregnancy being the likely cause, you should see your doctor immediately and ask him to refer you to the hospital because of your miscarriages. There, in all probability, you will be given some hormonal supplement in the early weeks of your pregnancy, to try and prevent a further miscarriage.

Internal examination

Q. I miscarried at eight weeks, earlier this year, after nearly 10 months of trying to conceive. (Yet with my first baby, who is now four, I became pregnant only the second time we tried.) What worries me is that just before I miscarried my doctor performed an internal check and a cervical smear—could this have caused the miscarriage? Also I have had a vaginal thrush infection on and off for the last two years which causes a heavy discharge—could this be responsible for my difficulty in becoming pregnant? What causes a miscarriage? Incidentally, I'm now keeping a temperature chart and it seems to show regular ovulation—but how long does it usually take for a normal woman to conceive?
Mrs. C.L., Notts.

A. A normal cervical smear test or an internal check could not possibly have caused a miscarriage. Around one third of miscarriages occur because the baby is implanted in the wrong site of the uterine wall, and another third because of some degree of foetal abnormality which is incompatible with growth. The remaining cases are often associated with a slight hormonal deficiency.
It is possible for an infection of thrush to impair your fertility. It does not affect it permanently, but whilst it is

present, particularly in view of the vaginal discharge it causes, it can make it difficult for sperm to pass through the cervix and fertilise the egg. However, once the infection is controlled, normal fertility returns.

The average time taken to conceive by a normal healthy couple is between one year and 18 months. Many women conceive easily with their first babies, but find it takes longer with later ones, and this is not by any means a sign of abnormality. The miscarriage would not have impaired your fertility, and I am sure that having demonstrated that you are ovulating regularly, it will only be a matter of time before you conceive again.

A tilted womb

Q. I think I have now had two miscarriages, and after the first one my doctor said that my womb pointed backwards. Could this have been the cause? The first time I'd missed a period for seven weeks and then when I started to bleed it was very heavy. I did not lose anything that looked much different—just a lot of clots —is this usual? Three months later and after the doctor's internal check up, it happened again—two missed periods and then a very painful and heavy period. I felt a bit nauseated before it all happened on the second occasion, and my breasts were sore too. How long now should I wait before trying again for a baby?
Mrs. C.J., Lincs.

A. With regard to your first miscarriage at seven weeks, the very small foetus would have been hard to distinguish from the clots which are passed in heavy menstrual bleeding.

The comment about a tilting womb was probably just a routine observation by your doctor. In fact, the uterus in a perfectly healthy woman can at times tilt backwards, forwards, or point upwards—its position frequently changing, often depending on the fullness of the bladder or rectum, and I would not, therefore, regard this as being at all significant. It would seem that it was a genuine miscarriage that you suffered some three months later, for the heavy period pains would have been caused by the uterus contracting to evacuate its contents. Without doing a pregnancy test, it is often very hard to distinguish whether a woman has in fact had a miscarriage or just a delayed and extra heavy period.

Having had two miscarriages, however, it would be sensible to allow yourself a period of six months or so before trying to conceive again, so that your periods can return to normal. Your hormones can then return to their natural levels, and when your body is faced once more with the challenge of conception, your chances of carrying it through normally will be enhanced.

Conflicting advice

Q. I've read quite a lot about miscarriage, and there seems to be conflicting advice on how long to wait, after a miscarriage, before trying to get pregnant again. What is your advice on this, and why? I've been particularly depressed and miserable since I miscarried. Is this usual?
Mrs. J.L., Lincs.

A. The reason many doctors recommend waiting three months is so that the first period can occur (at an unpredictable time) and will remove any retained products of conception that might have been left (it is often a little heavier than normal). The second period then occurs, often at a more predictable time, but not until the third period is it certain that the woman's menstruation has become regular. Regular periods show that a woman's hormonal profile has returned to normal and that she has probably started to ovulate again. Of course it is possible to conceive earlier than this, but if your body has gone through some hormonal 'shock' as a result of a miscarriage, you may miscarry again. There is certainly medical evidence to suggest that recurrent miscarriage occurs as the result of too frequent conceptions and for this reason the best policy is to wait for three periods before conceiving again. I do sympathise with your feelings of depression and distress after this miscarriage. Often such a depression is made worse by the hormonal changes, and I am certain that it is possible for a form of post-natal depression to occur after a miscarriage, as well as after a pregnancy.

Rubella dangers

Q. I was six weeks pregnant when I got German measles (I had not been immunised), and the following week I miscarried. I am consoled to think that perhaps nature knew what it was doing for I would have been terrified at the thought of a damaged baby. Could there have been some other cause though, and could the baby perhaps have been unharmed despite my illness?
Mrs. J.F., London NW3.

A. Your infection with German measles must have been responsible for the miscarriage, because this virus passes from the mother to the foetus and inevitably affects its development. From that point of view, there-fore, nature has, as you say, acted very wisely and I am quite sure that you need not feel that you lost an other-wise healthy baby through any other cause.

Conceived too soon?

Q. I miscarried, then conceived again before having a period—and now I'm very worried in case it was wrong to do this. Why are women recommended to wait before conceiving again? Also is it true—as someone told me—that if you get pregnant too soon you're more likely to have a handicapped baby?
Mrs. L.A., Cheshire.

A. I can appreciate your concern about having con-ceived so quickly after your previous miscarriage. The reason for making the standard suggestion to wait for three months is basically to ensure that the body returns to normal, and is ready to accept the hormonal chal-lenge of another pregnancy. However, if the body has recovered sufficiently to accept the challenge, pregnancy is possible, and in those circumstances, if the pregnancy is maintained, there is no need for anxiety. There is no evidence that there is a greater chance of giving birth to a handicapped child if it is conceived immediately after a miscarriage.

Still lactating

Q. Four weeks ago I lost my baby when I was 20 weeks pregnant. My doctor could offer me no real explanation, only that it was not my fault and would not happen again. How can he be so sure? From the time I was around three months pregnant I suffered with a low abdominal pain and low back ache, and at four months I started to lose blood and the flow gradually increased until I miscarried at five months. The loss of the baby has upset me greatly, and I have suffered with nerves and sleepless nights since. The doctor has given me some tranquillisers but I don't think I will feel normal again until I hold my next baby in my arms. Two days after my miscarriage I produced quite a supply of breast milk and still have some. Is this normal and will the milk go by itself?
Mrs. B.J., Norfolk.

A. It seems obvious that the foetus was implanted in a position in your uterus which was incompatible with survival to full term. It must have been very low down—perhaps near the cervix itself, and the baby was unable to survive. There is no reason for you to expect that this might happen again. Your body has gone through the normal hormonal changes of a pregnancy, and that is why you produced milk. Your doctor can prescribe tablets which will help to take this away. Most women who experience a miscarriage are likely to feel emotionally upset, and this can take many weeks and sometimes months to get over. There is no reason why, after a period of two or three months or so, you should not try for another baby, with every prospect of your next pregnancy being entirely normal.

Hormonal upset

Q.   I am 30, and three weeks ago I had a miscarriage at 12 weeks. After this I was given a D & C operation. We had been trying to have a baby for about two years from when I came off the pill. I have always had a fair amount of period pain, but in the last 18 months or so it has become almost unbearable. It now starts as early as 12 or 10 days before my period is due, with a dragging feeling in the pelvic area (not actually severe pain), backache, and my breasts are so sore they are almost unbearable to touch. I have to wear a 'sleep-bra' at night, and feel really miserable. I have been to my doctor about this and he said it was due to water retention and gave me some tablets to take each morning when required. I am afraid these did not help at all, so after a few months I went back to him and he gave me some pain-killing tablets. These did not help me either, so I gave up going. I have noticed my periods are getting much shorter now, lasting only one or two days. Could this have had anything to do with the miscarriage?
Mrs. M.A., Wilts.

A.   It certainly seems that a great deal of your menstrual difficulties are associated with hormonal irregularity, and your family doctor should refer you to a gynaecologist for advice and treatment. It will probably be necessary for you to take one of the hormonal supplements which, if carefully chosen, would certainly not affect your fertility.
It is always difficult to make a diagnosis at any distance, but it does seem suspicious that your miscarriage came after a period of hormonal insufficiency. I think, therefore, it would be fair to suspect that hormonal irregularity was the cause—or the most likely one at least—of the miscarriage itself.

Ageing factor

Q.   I am 41 years old, but unfortunately had a miscarriage at 11 weeks three weeks ago. I realise my age is against me, but my husband and I would very much like another child and so would be grateful for any help and advice. Although I understand it is early days yet, I want to know the course of action to take for the best possible result. Obviously we haven't too much time to spare. My questions are as follows:—

1) What is the cause of a miscarriage?
2) Can being tired, lifting and straining cause it?
3) How soon is it safe to try again?
4) Is there a danger in trying too soon?
5) How do I avoid another miscarriage?

We did not have intercourse from conception to miscarriage and only monthly before that. I married late, and my mother was 42 when I was born. 'Elderly' mums run in the family and this has always given me hope and encouragement.

Mrs. C.K., Scotland.

A. Miscarriage is a common occurrence at all ages with some 30 per cent, at least, of conceptions ending that way, and the causes are legion. Genetic abnormality of the foetus is probably the commonest, with inaccurate implantation, failure of the body to respond to the hormonal challenge of pregnancy and failure of development of the foetus beyond a certain stage being the other main reasons. In all these circumstances, therefore, although it is an old cliché, it is still true that miscarriage is nature's way of correcting its own mistakes. Therefore, lifting heavy weights, carrying things, anxiety and even insomnia have little part to play in what is a natural termination of a pregnancy.

The best time to try for a new pregnancy after a miscarriage is after three to six months. This period of time allows the body to return to its normal hormonal status. There is no actual danger in trying before that time, but if the body failed on the previous occasion to respond to the normal challenge of pregnancy and insufficient time is allowed to elapse for the hormones to return to normal, miscarriage is more likely with the second conception. There is virtually nothing that you can do to avoid a miscarriage once you have become pregnant— apart from avoiding excessive physical exertion. It is simply a matter of waiting to see for the first 12 weeks or so, whether the conception will develop successfully.

Nor is sexual intercourse harmful to a pregnancy.
It is most encouraging to learn that you are able to conceive, and you certainly have several years ahead of you in which you can still contemplate having children.

Private care

Q.   I have in the past year suffered two miscarriages (both between seven and a half and eight weeks). I have now not had a period for three months and know I must be pregnant again. I am seeing a gynaecologist but am very unhappy with his attitude. Every time I go there I seem to be faced with a 'couldn't care less' attitude. He keeps saying I have had only suspected miscarriages—although a foetus was produced both times. I have been refused hormone treatment, which he says does more harm than good, and can actually cause a miscarriage. In short, he is doing nothing positive at all. I had a pregnancy test taken at seven weeks (which was about 31 days after conception) which was negative. Now he says this is a bad sign, but wouldn't say why and hinted if I was really pregnant (and I'm not sure he thinks I am) then it must be dead. Despite all this he doesn't want to see me for another month.
Is this pregnancy test really the end as far as I'm concerned? I would have thought there must be some room for error. I have had a negative test at seven weeks before but I did subsequently miscarry.
What would you do in my situation? I feel like complaining officially because of the indifferent treatment I seem to get, as though I'm not really important at all. Could you tell me also if he is right and the foetus is already dead, how long would it be before it came away and should I do anything?
Mrs. E.S., Hants.

A.   It may of course be that your gynaecologist is not able to be precise with regard to his predictions, and the fact that you have had a negative pregnancy test does tend to suggest in any case that there is very little in terms of practical treatment that could be done. Pregnancy tests are not totally reliable, and in some cases the amount of hormones in a pregnant woman's urine is insufficient for the test to react. However, this in itself does not necessarily indicate that hormone supplements would help.

I know how disappointing it must be for you, particularly to be told not to return for at least another month, but regrettably there is not very much else that could be done. It may well be that you have conceived and that the foetus is implanted in a place in the uterus that is incompatible with further development. Due to a temporary hormonal irregularity the period that would otherwise have come has been delayed, and whilst it is perhaps rather harsh (if technically accurate) to tell a woman that this means that the foetus is dead, it might have been more helpful if it had been explained that this is a possibility. I am afraid you will have to wait and see what happens over the next month. If you are going to miscarry it will happen within the next month.

It cannot be denied that patients are sometimes treated with indifference, perhaps because of pressure of work, but the only way round that is to go for private care (which can be expensive). You could ask your family doctor to refer you to another gynaecologist as a private patient, if only for one or two private consultations, and you would certainly then find that the specialist would concentrate on answering all your questions.

No help

Q.   I am writing in the hope that you will give me some honest and detailed advice which my doctor seems unable or unwilling to give me.

Just under a fortnight ago I suffered my second miscarriage (the first was four months earlier). Both terminated at approximately eight weeks at the expected time of my second period. I was particularly upset this second time, as I am convinced that my doctor could have helped me.

When I contacted him, all I had was a brown discharge with no pains at all. I had just had a pregnancy test (taken at just under seven weeks). This was negative, and because of this he refused to visit me at home. I was told if I really thought it was necessary I would have to attend the surgery. I stayed in bed all day and saw him on a Tuesday evening. The discharge in his own words was 'nothing to worry about'. He examined me and then just said it was a delayed period and did nothing. Nothing I said had any effect. My periods are never three days late, let alone three weeks. Two days later I miscarried. He did come to see me after this but neither apologised nor said anything helpful other than that the baby must have been dead for about a week or so!

Just how easy is it to prevent an early miscarriage once a loss begins? This same doctor also told me that hormone treatment normally does little good and that the general medical opinion was that it was of little use. Is this really true?

I was told I could see a gynaecologist, but I have heard nothing since it happened.

Mrs. C.B., Lancs.

A. It does seem that it has been a lack of necessary hormones that was responsible for your pregnancies not continuing after conception, and this would be supported by the evidence of the negative pregnancy test. Since a positive result depends on finding sufficient hormones in the urine, the implication is obviously that there were not enough circulating in your bloodstream for the pregnancy to be maintained. In such circumstances, once a vaginal loss begins, there is really very little that can be done to prevent a miscarriage. In your case, I do feel that appropriate hormone treatment as soon as your period becomes overdue again is going to be the answer. I disagree with your general practitioner, for it is, in fact, a generally held medical opinion that for the woman who demonstrates a clear hormonal insufficiency, hormonal supplements are the most sensible and hopeful form of treatment.

You should ask your doctor to make sure that you are referred to a gynaecologist firstly for a check-up, in view of your two miscarriages and, secondly, for advice as to what should be done whenever you next conceive. In this way you will have access to a specialist immediately your next period is overdue, and once a pregnancy is confirmed then your specialist will start the appropriate treatment for you.

You will need a period of rest to allow your body to return to normal, and I strongly suggest that you do not try to conceive for at least a further six months. Only then, if your menstrual cycle has completely returned to normal and you have had at least three normal and consecutive menstrual periods, should you start a baby again.

Placental revelation

Q. I am 27, and seven weeks ago I lost my baby when I was 24 weeks pregnant. I knew right from the start there was something wrong, and was worried the whole time. Can worry cause a miscarriage? The doctor said the afterbirth was a bit small, and that they thought it wasn't attached properly.
Mrs. D.F., Wales.

A. Anxiety and worry cannot cause miscarriage, and from what you tell me it seems that the cause in your case was the insufficient development of the afterbirth. This can occur quite commonly when the afterbirth is not implanted in the correct place on the wall of the womb, although other causes such as high blood pressure, hormonal deficiency and some degree of foetal abnormality due to a genetic accident, can also be responsible. It is, however, a very rare occurrence, and for that reason you can confidently look forward to future pregnancies being in all probability, entirely normal.

Suspicious infection

Q. After losing two babies at seven months it was diagnosed that the neck of my womb was weak and during my third pregnancy a Shirodkar stitch was inserted. As a result I gave birth to a little boy two years ago. Because I had a Caesarean section the consultant left the stitch in, but said if I didn't have another child within two years it would have to be removed. When the stitch was inserted I started having a very heavy discharge which continued after the baby was born. About six months ago the discharge became dark and smelly and the doctor gave me antibiotics to clear up the infection. However, although the dark colour is no longer evident, the discharge makes me wet and sore. I need to have a bath every morning and I have to wear a sanitary pad all the time. My husband finds that he is sore and itchy after intercourse. We have been trying for a baby for the past year. We never had any problems in conceiving before. Also my periods are irregular (about one every two months) and very heavy, and although I have not changed my diet or lifestyle I have put on a stone in weight in the last three months. I have tried to talk to my doctor about all this, but he only has time to write prescriptions and makes me feel as though I am wasting his time. Ideally I would like to see the consultant I was originally under but I can't seem to get past my doctor.

Mrs. W.M., Yorks.

A.   The problems you are experiencing certainly suggest that you are in need once more of skilled gynaecological advice. The discharge should not be continuing in this way, and the fact that your husband is also affected suggests that you may well be infected with a thrush-like organism. A thorough investigation and gynaecological assessment is called for, and I suspect that removal of the Shirodkar suture will be necessary. You and your husband should ask your doctor very clearly to be referred back to your gynaecologist for an assessment. If you feel financially able to do so you might even suggest that you would be prepared to go privately (which would cost around perhaps £20 to £30). Certainly you should not put up with the continual discharge and soreness which you have at the moment, and this condition will without doubt inhibit your chances of conceiving. It will be necessary, therefore, for this matter to be completely cleared up before you are likely to become pregnant again.

Fibroid untreated

Q. I had an X-ray at the hospital to investigate a queried incompetent cervix after a miscarriage at 20 weeks. The miscarriage was 18 months ago. I understood at the time that a weak cervix was probably the cause, but my concern is that I have not yet become pregnant again.

The X-ray showed weakness in the internal opening and a fibroid or polyp in the cervix. The doctor said he would put a stitch in to tighten the cervix and investigate and possibly remove the fibroid. In the X-ray it was visible but wasn't much of an obstruction. Could either of these things be preventing conception? Is it usual for a stitch to be inserted before a pregnancy? What is a fibroid and why should I have one? I am 36 and we very much want children.

Mrs. T.S., London.

A. The investigations which revealed a fibroid and a polyp do suggest that these should be dealt with before another conception—for the presence of polyps, with the excessive cervical secretion which they usually initiate, reduces fertility. Fibroids can also reduce the amount of space for the developing foetus in the womb, and thus cause problems not only with conception but with the successful completion of a pregnancy. A fibroid is basically just an overgrowth of the fibrous tissue (that of course is how it gets its name) that exists within the muscular layer of the uterus. They are perfectly simple and entirely non-malignant and really should be seen as little overgrowths of scar tissue and nothing more. They occur in nearly all women, and more commonly in those over 30.

You should return to the specialist as soon as possible and ask for their removal, particularly in view of your age. Although you are by no means anywhere near the end of your reproductive life, I am sure you will appreciate that conceptions occur less easily for the older woman than for the younger one. Finally, with regard to the incompetent cervix, I cannot really believe that your doctor intends to stitch this up prior to your becoming pregnant and you may have misunderstood this. The 'purse string suture' is usually done after a pregnancy has been confirmed, maintaining a closed off uterine cavity for the developing foetus, reducing the risk of a miscarriage occurring as the foetus grows. The stitch is removed when labour starts.

Infection

Q. I had an abortion when I was 20 which resulted in a haemorrhage and a D & C being done at the local hospital. I also had an infection which had to be cleared up with quite a lot of antibiotics. Obviously the doctor who induced the abortion had only broken my waters and left nature to work by itself, resulting in the infection as I only started feeling pains two days later and had to be rushed into hospital. What I would like to know is, firstly, whether this has prevented us from having any more children, as we have now been trying for quite a while to no avail and, secondly, whether this abortion could have closed up my tubes. A couple of weeks after I had the D & C, a gynaecologist examined me and said that all was O.K., which I suppose meant that I no longer had any infection. My husband and I have a regular and normal sex life and yet I still cannot conceive. I have normal periods without too much bother, and they usually last about four or five days. I am sure I am releasing an egg every month as I have taken my temperature every morning, so the conclusion we have come to is that my abortion must have prevented me having another child.
Mrs. T.L., Jersey.

A. The average time taken for a healthy couple to achieve conception is anything between six and 18 months, once they are taking account of the woman's fertile period by keeping a temperature chart. It may well be that you are becoming too anxious, too soon, and you should allow this period of time to elapse before seeking advice from a specialist. If, however, this period of time has already elapsed, you should arrange for both of you to be examined by a specialist in infertility, who will carry out appropriate tests on both of you. These will include one called the gas insufflation test which will, in combination with an X-ray of your uterine tubes when a radio-opaque dye has been inserted, show quite clearly whether there is any possibility of tubal abnormality or obstruction having resulted from the infection you had following the abortion. There are, however, no grounds in your letter for assuming that this has happened and, whilst it is sensible to bear it in mind as a possibility, it is no more than that until the appropriate test proves otherwise.

When is it safe?

Q.   How long after a miscarriage must we wait before we have intercourse? I lost heavily for a week, but it has stopped now. My husband uses sheaths. Should I rest in any special way having lost a baby (it was only six weeks) and how long will it be before my periods are back to normal?
Mrs. P.B., Lancs.

A.   It is perfectly all right for you and your husband to have intercourse whenever you wish, now that you have stopped bleeding. There is no necessity for any more rest than you find normal, and it is most likely that your next period will come around four weeks or so from the onset of your miscarriage, although in some cases it can take a little longer for the normal menstrual cycle to be resumed.

Understandable misery

Q.   Please help me—it's four months now since I went into labour (I was overdue) and my baby was born dead. I cry every night and whenever I see any of my friends with their babies I cross the street to avoid them. I've refused to visit my husband's sister because she has two babies under four. My husband makes it worse by fussing over everyone he knows who has children—he seems to make a special point of playing with the neighbours' children, and when I watch him I feel

terrible and burst into tears. How long will it be before
I'm pregnant again?
Mrs. W.G., Scotland.

A.   I can assure you that the feelings you describe are
perfectly normal for a woman who has gone through
what you have. There is inevitably a depressive reaction
to any grief, made worse of course by the hormonal
changes that occur after a pregnancy. Somehow it is
easier if it is a miscarriage than a stillbirth, because you
have not carried the baby so long, but even then there
can be an awful and upsetting let-down. It is natural that
every baby you see will remind you of your loss. If you
can force yourself to be in contact with other people's
babies, you may well be brought to tears many times—
and there is nothing wrong with that, but it will help
you to adjust as time passes. There is one very important
fact for you to remember and that is that you have
proved your fertility—you can have babies—and even
though you are not yet pregnant again, it will not be too
long before you are, probably within six to nine months.
Because of your history, there need be no fear of a
recurrence of your tragedy, as plans will be made for
the earliest intervention by way of bringing on labour if
there is the slightest sign of any problems near term.
Finally, I think your husband is in a way trying to help
you when he fusses with other people's babies; you
should join him in doing so and you may find it relaxes
your own tensions and anxieties by playing mother—
even though it will be very hurtful at first.

CHAPTER IV
Fertility, Drugs & Insemination

How effective

Q.   My husband and I have been trying unsuccessfully for a baby for about 18 months. Last month I saw a gynaecologist, and he prescribed Clomiphene tablets, two per day for five days. Apparently I was not ovulating. I have now taken one course of Clomiphene, and my temperature mid-month took over three days to rise to its top level, and then went up even more just before my period was due.
Could you tell me just how effective these fertility drugs are, and by how much the temperature is supposed to rise? We are both a bit fed up with keeping these charts, which we have done for over a year now. I am due to take another course of Clomiphene, the same dosage, next month. Am I more likely to conceive twins when taking several courses of this drug?
Mrs. T.C., Hamps.

A.   Clomiphene is one of the most effective and best-tried fertility drugs. As you have only taken one course of these tablets, you must wait a little longer before drawing any conclusions with regard to its effect. Nevertheless, even on the one course you did have a mid-cycle rise in your daily temperature and this is encouraging, suggesting that ovulation may well be effectively stimulated already. The normal temperature dip and rise for a woman who is not taking one of the stimulant drugs, is over 48 hours or so, but where there has been some difficulty with ovulating in the past, this temperature rise will be a little more prolonged, as in your case. You must continue to keep the temperature chart, even though it is tedious, for this is really the only way in which the effectiveness of the drug (apart, of course, from conception) can be assessed. As to the likelihood of multiple conceptions, this is always a possibility with the ovulatory stimulant drugs, but it is less common nowadays than when these drugs first became available. The incidence of twins (and more) being conceived is not associated with the duration of time for which these drugs are taken, but rather with the dosage. Gradually, infertility specialists have gained a great deal of knowledge about the right dosage of these fairly powerful drugs, and it is preferable to use small doses for long periods of time rather than to use, as used to be done, very high dosages for just one or two months. In a large survey of closely monitored patients who took Clomiphene, there were only seven per cent who had twins, 0.5 per cent triplets, and 0.3 per cent quadruplets. So you can be reassured that it is perfectly safe for you to continue to take it for quite some time, perhaps even for a year or two or longer if necessary, without running any special risk of a multiple pregnancy.

Four already

Q.   I had great difficulty in conceiving my last child. I consulted a doctor who advised me to take a few courses of the fertility drug Clomiphene and I became pregnant a few months later.
I have four children, the youngest of whom is seven months, and the oldest is eight. I should like to complete my family as I am now 30, and should like to know what my chances of becoming pregnant are likely to be. Will I have to take the drugs again in order to boost my fertility? I used the temperature method to find my ovulation time, but as yet, having had intercourse on the

relevant days, have not had any success. Please advise me as to any methods—other than the temperature method, that tell when ovulation takes place? My cycle varies from 24-29 days.
Mrs. S.C., Bucks.

A. It is reassuring to note that after treatment with Clomiphene you became pregnant and also, having given birth to four children your fertility is not in any doubt. In view of the fact that your youngest baby is still only seven months old, your opportunities of conceiving since then have been few (probably less than four or five in view of the quite frequent suppression of ovulation after a pregnancy) and I would not, therefore, suggest that you have any cause for anxiety as yet about your present failure to conceive.
The most useful suggestion I can make, therefore, is that you continue to use your temperature chart to detect ovulation time and persist for another six to nine months or so, before seeking any further help. There is no more reliable method of finding your fertile period than keeping a temperature chart.

What next?

Q. I have been treated over the past five years for infertility. I already have children, the youngest of whom is two. We have been trying for a year and a half for another baby, but without success. Before my last baby was born I was treated with Clomiphene for three months, following the usual tests—insufflation of the tubes, sperm tests for my husband, and so on.
After my last baby when we again had difficulties, I went to a gynaecologist who started me on Clomiphene tablets—one at first for five days and then he increased the dosage to two. I have now finished six months' treatment and still I am not pregnant. I have been recording my morning temperature and although I noticed a temperature difference in the first four charts, it appears that I did not ovulate for the last two cycles. I don't understand how this could happen as Clomiphene is supposed to stimulate ovulation.

My doctor also had a prolactin test performed and said the result was 'favourable'. Would you tell me what this test indicates, and what 'favourable' might suggest? Also, what further treatment is available for a person with my complaint? I might add that I am 30 years old—my husband is 38.
Mrs. H.R., Scotland.

A.   The prolactin test is to detect the level in the bloodstream of a hormone called prolactin, which, if present in excess, suppresses ovulation. Your favourable test, therefore, indicated a low level and this is reassuring.
Having taken a course of Clomiphene, it is likely that the next course of action will be to suspend all treatment for a period of between three to six months and then to recommence the ovulatory stimulant drug in order to obtain a more beneficial effect. This may be frustrating for you, but the object is to prevent the body becoming accustomed to fertility stimulant drugs and resisting their effect as would certainly seem to have occurred in your case from the evidence of your temperature charts. Like all forms of biochemical stimulus, the effect of Clomiphene can wear off after a time, and the resistance of the ovaries to its stimulation can increase if it is persisted with for too long. However, provided a sufficient period of time is allowed to elapse after a course of the drug, this resistance fades away, and when medication is renewed, the original highly effective stimulation returns.

Am I a freak?

Q.   I had my first four children with little difficulty, but I had a difficult time conceiving my last baby. I went to a gynaecologist after two and a half years of trying, and he did a salpingography, which showed that the tubes were open. He then gave me a course of Clomiphene, and after three courses I conceived.
After my last baby was born my periods did not start for six months, and only then after a further course of Clomiphene. All went well for three months but then my periods stopped for another three months. I again took

Clomiphene for a few months but failed to conceive. My temperature chart indicated that I ovulated while taking it, and I had intercourse at the appropriate time but still failed to conceive. My specialist then put me on a 40-day course of Bromocryptine, but I failed to ovulate.

I now find that my last period is overdue by 15 days, but a pregnancy test was negative when my period was 12 days overdue. One of my breasts has been tender for the past three weeks. I don't know what to think. The test says I am not pregnant but where has the period gone? At my last visit to my specialist, I asked if he would do a laparoscopy, but he refused. I cannot understand how my whole menstrual cycle has become so disrupted as I never had trouble before my last child.

I have become very depressed about the matter and only wish to return to normal or else find out by examination what is wrong and not to keep taking tablets every time I want to become pregnant. Am I a freak for wanting more babies? I'm 39 at the end of this year.

Mrs. S.M., Midlands.

A.   It is possible that you are pregnant, but a negative pregnancy test when a period is less than 14 days overdue is not particularly reliable. Indeed, because of the breast tenderness it could easily be that the negative test is wrong, but your doctors will arrange for another one if your next expected period fails to arrive. However, because of your previous history of menstrual irregularity and treatment with various hormonal supplements in order to stimulate ovulation, you must be prepared for the fact that a delayed period in your case may not necessarily mean that you are pregnant.

Your doctor's refusal to perform a laparoscopy is very reasonable, for surgical interference with the abdominal or pelvic organs in the early weeks of pregnancy is not to be recommended. Your recent menstrual irregularity is a quite common experience and not one to become too depressed or anxious about. Of course you are not a freak for wanting more children when you already have five, for a generation or so ago, you would have been considered strange for only having five when our grandparents so commonly had nine, 10 and many more.

With regard to your age, it is worth emphasising that since the average age of the onset of the menopause is nowadays around 48, there is plenty of time for you to have many more children, and if this is what you want, you will receive all the help that may be necessary.

Lastly, whilst I understand your current enthusiasm and anxiety for conceiving, if it does prove that you have not become pregnant, you might consider a period of a year or two without drugs in order to allow your body's hormones to return to their normal level, and to allow ovulation to take place more naturally and be less affected by ovulatory stimulants. I say this because very occasionally excessive use of ovulatory stimulants can lead to a certain kind of 'ovary exhaustion' and ultimately in the long run work to produce the opposite effect from that desired. Similarly, anxiety and excessive concern about wishing to conceive, can in itself sometimes act as a fertility suppressant.

How long

Q. I had a baby boy four years ago, and then my periods stopped (they have always been irregular). I saw a consultant three or four times, had X-rays, blood and urine tests and then was prescribed Bromocryptine last year.
Can you tell me what this drug is for—and how long I have to take it?
Mrs. S.E., London.

A. Bromocryptine is prescribed for women who are infertile because of an excess of prolactin, as it suppresses production of this hormone. Bromocryptine can be very effective in allowing ovulation to take place. It is frequently necessary to take it for quite a long period of time, until ovulation has been shown to be taking place, and a pregnancy has begun. This can only be done, however, if all the regular tests are undertaken and the results are reassuring.

The regime of treatment is that the Bromocryptine must be stopped as soon as the pregnancy is confirmed because a certain amount of the hormone prolactin is necessary for the successful continuation of the pregnancy, and to artificially suppress it for too long, or in too excessive a dosage, would obviously be harmful.

Time to stop

Q.   We've been trying for a baby for three years, and everything's been done but my specialist now wants to stop my fertility drugs. I'm on Clomiphene and Bromocryptine, and I feel desperate because I have been told I can only have them for another three months. Is there anything stronger I could have? I can't understand why I'm not pregnant—all the tests on both me and my husband were normal. We will be 30 in 2 years' time. What can we do?
Mrs. T.S., Wilts.

A.   It is encouraging to learn that you have had all the appropriate tests at the sub-fertility clinic and that you have been on both Clomiphene tablets to stimulate ovulation and also on Bromocryptine to reduce your prolactin level. Your despair at feeling that the time limit set for medication is running out, is understandable. Even though you will be finishing the course, it could easily be that their use has semi-permanently lowered your secretion rate of prolactin and led to some ovulatory stimulant effect, and there is no reason, therefore, why you should not conceive at some time in the future.
There are no stronger fertility drugs than the ones you have had, but it may be that your specialists will put you back on another course of treatment in time. The most reassuring feature of your investigation is that your husband has a normal sperm count, and that you have been shown to have no gynaecological abnormality. At the same time, you should bear in mind that anxiety and worry may have played a part, too. In fact, there is fairly recent medical evidence that prolactin levels rise when a person is worried and anxious, and that explains why so often, after a couple have almost given up hope of ever actually conceiving, and in particular a wife becomes resigned to being childless—this resignation

and relaxation causes a drop in the secretion of many of her hormones—particularly those associated with anxiety, and a consequent lowering of the prolactin level.

I can appreciate how tense you must feel, but you are both still young, and I am sure that you will appreciate that you have at least some 15 to 20 years of fertile life ahead of you, and you need have very little doubt that you will ultimately conceive.

IUD removal

Q.   I have an intra-uterine device fitted, and we want to start a family next year—we're both 25. What advice would you give me with regard to having my coil out and starting a family?
Mrs. M.H., Hants.

A.   It would be advisable to have the IUD removed three months before trying to conceive in order to allow any chronic irritation of the uterine cavity caused by the IUD's presence, to settle down. I would suggest therefore, that you have the device removed, allow at least two normal periods to occur on their own, and then try to become pregnant. Naturally, it may take a little while before you conceive, although many couples, particularly if they are young and healthy, do succeed in the first few months after stopping all forms of contraception.

Problems after IUD

Q.   Four years ago, after the birth of our second son, I decided to have an IUD. I had this removed seven months ago, thinking I would become pregnant straight away, planning that the birth of a new baby and my younger son's commencing school would coincide. I was not told by my doctor that I would not conceive straight away—otherwise I would have had it removed sooner to allow for this. The thing that really concerns me is that I'm sure I do conceive but my body is continuing to reject it, as it did when a 'foreign body' was

present in the womb. I usually have regular periods, but when I think I conceive I have some symptoms of pregnancy (more pronounced than pre-menstrual symptoms) and my period comes a week late, either preceded or followed by a 'clot'. Clotting also used to occur when the IUD was present. Could you please tell me if this generally happens after an IUD and give me some indication of how long it goes on? Four years is a long time and perhaps my body has become 'trained' to behave in this way. (I am 29).
Mrs. B.T., Avon.

A.   It seems that you are still experiencing the after-effects of chronic irritation of the uterine wall, and you might well have had one or two miscarriages as a result of this. Ask your doctor to arrange for you to see a gynaecologist, for, in all probability, curettage (D & C operation) of the uterus is necessary in order to clear away any chronically inflamed material that might be there. This fairly simple operation will not involve you in being admitted to hospital for longer than 24 hours at the most, but it will clear up all your problems and difficulties. Once this is done, you will be able to go ahead planning for a pregnancy. It will not be too long before you conceive—the fertility of you and your husband is not in any doubt.

Coil and hormonal problems

Q.   After the birth of my last baby I had a coil fitted, and at first it was fine, and gave no trouble, but 12 months later, my periods began being troublesome, heavy and irregular. I saw my doctor who said that a woman's menstrual cycle goes through periods of change and that it would right itself. I had the coil 12 months later as I was told this would help, but it didn't. I had various medicines which didn't help either, and all the while, my periods were getting worse, leaving me only a few days in the month when I wasn't bleeding, plus the irritability of pre-menstrual tension. At the beginning of this year I went on the pill to help, but it made no difference. Finally, I saw a specialist who said it was all to do with my hormones and put me on hormone pills for three months. They were called Primolut, and they did help a lot. I finished them two months ago.

Now we would like another baby. However, about a week before my period is due, I start getting an offensive discharge. It continues until a couple of days before the period starts. My doctor says it is decaying blood which is why it is offensive and nothing can be done about it. Will this stop me conceiving?

Mrs. F.K., Devon.

A. There is little doubt that your coil caused a great deal of uterine irritation, and that in the end it took the hormone tablets to right the abnormality. However, things are not yet quite back to normal, and you still need the supervision of the specialist in order to overcome the pre-menstrual losses you mention.

You will probably find that it takes quite a while for you to conceive in view of the duration of the hormonal upset. Moreover, if your menstrual disorder is not corrected, then you may well be exposed to an increased risk of a miscarriage if conception were to take place. You can be reassured by the fact that the medication worked so well for you last time—it will again, and it will probably not be long before you conceive.

Pregnant with an IUD

Q. I have a Copper 7 IUD in place and yet it has been confirmed that I am pregnant. How could this happen? Will I miscarry? My doctor is arranging a scan for me, to see where the IUD is, but I thought I'd need an X-ray.

Mrs. C.J., Bucks.

A. Conception can occur despite the use of an IUD, for the IUD works by preventing implantation of the foetus, not fertilisation of the egg, which occurs in the fallopian tube. Whilst it is remarkably successful as a form of fertility control, there is a pregnancy rate of one in 2000. There is a tendency for miscarriage to occur slightly more frequently in these pregnancies, but if it is going to occur it usually tends to do so in the first 12 weeks. Once that stage has been passed without a miscarriage, one can assume that the placenta is developing in an unobstructed way, and that the foetal growth is proceeding normally. An ultrasound scan can detect the IUD wherever it might be, even if it is buried in the afterbirth, and because of the presence of copper wire, an X-ray can be a much more effective way of diagnosing its presence. Nevertheless, as I am sure you will appreciate, the use of X-rays in early pregnancy is not recommended unless there is some vital reason and I would have thought that the scan which your doctor has suggested would be adequate. It is possible to continue a perfectly successful pregnancy with an IUD in place, if the tests show that the foetus and the placenta are unimpaired by its presence.

Remove it or carry on?

Q.   I am 10 weeks pregnant and conceived with a coil fitted (Copper 7). The FP clinic said it wouldn't harm the foetus but wanted to remove it. Surely that is a contradiction? Anyway, as it happened the threads weren't visible and they said it would be under the placenta or it may have been expelled at some stage. They have also informed my doctor that it could be an ectopic pregnancy.
I am worried what effect this will have on my baby.
Mrs. J.A., Norfolk.

A.   I can well understand your anxiety and concern, and there really are only two possible courses of action. One is the removal of the IUD and the possibility of the pregnancy itself being terminated, should the IUD be inextricably involved with either the placenta or the foetus's membrane. The second is to leave the IUD in place and allow the pregnancy to continue which will entail periodic investigation by ultrasound scan to ensure that the foetus is developing normally despite the presence of the IUD, and it is really for you to decide. Had the pregnancy been ectopic, the matter would, of course, inevitably have solved itself by now, as at 10 weeks, a tubal pregnancy is too large to be symptomless.

If you do decide to allow the pregnancy to continue, it would be reassuring for you to know that there are several hundred babies born each year perfectly normally and entirely unharmed, despite the presence of an IUD in the uterus at the same time.

Donors—who and how?

Q. Where do doctors get the donors from, when artificial insemination is performed, and how precisely is it done?
Mrs. G.A., Berks.

A. The anonymity of the donor is always considered to be essential, and the semen is frequently obtained from healthy young medical students. They may be paid a small fee (£2 or so) and produce the specimen not more than two hours before the patient is seen by the specialist. A woman needing this procedure (because her husband is totally sterile or has had a vasectomy for example) would keep an ovulation chart, and at the expected time of her maximum fertility, arrange an appointment with the gynaecologist. He would insert the semen through a syringe into her cervix, and after lying still for 30 minutes or so, she would be allowed home. The process might have to be repeated each month for several months before conception occurred.

"Do it yourself" insemination

Q. Some time during the last year, I read about it being possible for a husband and wife to carry out artificial insemination at home using the husband's semen. Is this true, and if so, would you give me details of how to go about it?
Mrs. K.M., Wales.

A. The method which you have heard about is where the husband produces a sample of seminal fluid, which is ejaculated into the cup of a cervical cap or diaphragm, and this is then carefully inserted into the vagina by the wife so that it is held in place against the cervix. The purpose is to ensure that the seminal fluid is kept in contact with the cervix (and, therefore, the entrance to the womb) for as long as possible in the hope that the spermatozoa will find it easier to penetrate the cervical mucus, and proceed up through the womb and achieve fertilisation of an egg cell. This do-it-yourself method has to be co-ordinated with a very carefully kept temperature chart in order to determine a woman's date of ovulation, and the method has to be used on several consecutive occasions after ovulation has occurred if there is to be any hope of success.

It is not as efficient as the standard medical method of artificial insemination using the husband's sperm, for then the seminal fluid is, in fact, injected into the cervix and up into the uterus. It does have the advantage, however, that it can be carried out at home without embarrassment and intervention of any other person. I would suggest you ask your local Family Planning Clinic to provide a cervical cap or diaphragm, temperature charts and a thermometer and so on, and relevant detailed instructions.

Sperm rejection?

Q. Three years ago I became pregnant after seven years of treatment, and I was told that I had been rejecting my husband's sperm. We have been trying for another baby since our son was born. Last time I had to have artificial insemination using my husband's sperm. Will I need it again—or will I have stopped rejecting his sperm by now?
Mrs. B.K., Northants.

A. There is no reason why you should not receive the same assistance as you had before after a reasonable period of time of trying to become pregnant in the normal way. If you had developed antibodies to your husband's sperm, causing you to reject its fertilising properties, then your pregnancy may well have neutralised these antibodies and you could easily be now in a state where there is, in fact, no rejection taking place at all. You should attempt to conceive for the next year or so in the normal way, and then if you are not successful, ask your doctor to refer you again to the specialist.

Vasectomy problems

Q. Is artificial insemination only for the childless? My husband who was married before, has had a vasectomy and was told it could not be reversed. He has two sons by his first wife, but we'd dearly love a family that we could bring up together. How can we go about it?
Mrs. S.A., Oxon.

A. Conceiving by means of artificial insemination is not restricted to childless women at all, but would be available for any woman whose husband was incapable of inseminating her himself.
Obviously as a result of your husband's vasectomy, this applies to you and I am sure that if you are both quite certain that this is the right step to take, your family doctor can refer you to the appropriate specialist for this kind of help.
You are quite right in your assumption that vasectomy is almost irreversible, and certainly any hopes of restoring your husband's fertility this way should not really be entertained, firstly because there are so few specialists in the country undertaking this form of operation and secondly, because when it has been tried, the results in terms of restored fertility have been quite dismal. For that reason, therefore, artificial insemination is the only possibility open to you.

Seminal problems

Q. Could there be something wrong with my husband's semen? It's yellow and sometimes has flecks of blood in it. He's older than me (he's 38) and we haven't had any children yet as we have only been married three months. Should anything be done about this?
Mrs. F.B., Midlands.

A. If there was anything at all abnormal with your husband's seminal fluid or spermatozoa, then conception would not occur. The condition that you mention is caused by varicose veins in the scrotum and around the testicles. When this occurs, as it often does in older men, there is sometimes some discolouration of the seminal fluid. This, in itself, is of no significance, but nevertheless, your husband should ask your doctor for an examination to ensure that all is well, and then arrange for a series of three semen analysis tests to be carried out. As a result of these, any treatment or further investigations necessary will then be undertaken for both of you.

Will I ever have his baby?

Q. What is involved in a vasectomy? Does it alter a man—sexually, I mean? I'm divorced but likely to marry a man who's had a vasectomy and would like to know more about this operation—could I ever become pregnant by him?

A. The vasectomy operation is a relatively simple one. A small part of the tube which leads from the testicles to the urethra and, therefore, carries the spermatozoa during ejaculation, is removed. The man, therefore, continues to ejaculate a certain amount of seminal fluid, but this does not contain any of the sperm cells which can lead to fertilisation. The normal secretions of male sex hormones are taking place in the testicles, so the 'maleness' of the individual is unaffected, and there is no effect on the nervous system or the enjoyment of a normal sex life afterwards. A man who has had a vasectomy is infertile, and there would be no possibility of having his children.

Vasectomy reversal?

Q. Can a vasectomy be reversed? I've read an American article about transplants of the cut-away tube being put in. What would be the conditions under which it would be undertaken?
Mrs. G.B., Surrey.

A. Attempts to reverse vasectomies have proved very unsuccessful. Only very rarely has it been done in special social circumstances (for example premature death of former wife or children) and even then the results have almost invariably been disappointing. Reports that you may have read about the success of attempts in America to replace the sperm canal with tube implants have been somewhat exaggerated. Vasectomy should be regarded as irreversible.

What happened?

Q. This is my second marriage and my husband has had his vasectomy reversed. In the last year I was pregnant on two occasions but on both of them I miscarried and now, after a recent test, my husband's sperm count is reported as nil. What can have happened to him? The surgeon who reversed the vasectomy has said nothing more can be done—should we get another opinion? Will I get pregnant again do you think?
Mrs. D.J., London.

A. I was most interested to learn that in your present marriage you were able to conceive even though your husband had previously had a vasectomy which had been reversed. It is very sad to learn that, despite this, you then miscarried on two occasions, for a reversal operation after a vasectomy is seldom successful.
However, in view of your husband's recent negative sperm tests it certainly does suggest that there has been some closure of the tubes, despite the repair. This may well have been brought about by the developing of scar tissue and the likelihood, therefore, of you becoming pregnant in the future is remote.
The surgical advice which your husband has already had is quite correct, for there is a limit to the amount of surgery which can be done in such a small area of the body without the complications of further scar tissue developing. There would be very few surgeons who would be prepared to undertake a second attempt at reversal.

CHAPTER V

Next Baby—When?

No second baby

Q. We have been trying for a second baby for 14 months now. I have been to my doctor twice about it; the first time he advised me to keep a temperature chart for about five months, which showed that I was ovulating; the second time, we just had a long talk, and he told us to keep trying for another four months and to return then if I was not pregnant, when he would do some tests.

It took me nine months to conceive our son, who is now two years old. I am now feeling really depressed about the whole thing. I don't think I can stand any more of this, and the thought of having to be examined to see if there is anything the matter with me, depresses me even more. I would like to point out that my doctor asked if my husband would have a sperm count test, but he said no, definitely not, so please could you suggest anything?

Mrs. S.P., Oxon.

A. With second conceptions it can take as long as a year or 18 months or so for the average, healthy woman to conceive. The great majority (at least 99 per cent) however, do eventually successfully conceive a second, third and fourth child.

It is a pity that your husband is not prepared to co-operate with a sperm count test. Perhaps he might change his mind at some time in the future. It might well be helpful for both of you to plan a specific interval during which you will continue to try to conceive, and after which you will ask your family doctor to refer you to a gynaecologist for any investigations which might be considered necessary.

I suggest that you allow another six months to go by, and by then (for it will then have been 20 months since you started trying to become pregnant) your husband might have changed his mind about the tests, and you might feel much more reconciled to them. I assure you that they are always done tactfully and understandingly and, seeing that their object is to achieve any possible treatment which might be necessary to help a couple to conceive, you will appreciate how worthwhile they are.

Why three sperm tests?

Q.   We do so want another baby, and we've both had all the tests and been told everything's all right. We've been trying now for over a year (our daughter was conceived after only two months), but there are still some things I'm very worried about. I'm booked for a laparoscopy next month. What happens when this is done—and if I did get pregnant this time, would it make me miscarry? My husband also had to have three sperm tests. Why was this? Does it mean something's wrong? Incidentally, the last test had to be done on the day my temperature chart showed I'd ovulated which was a real inconvenience.
Mrs. A.Mc., Glasgow.

A.   The laparoscopy would be delayed or cancelled if you were pregnant. If you were not the procedure would be quite simple. It is a visual inspection of the internal pelvic organs through a very tiny fibre optic tube. This is inserted via a small incision just below the navel to permit the surgeon to look at the ovaries and the internal organs to make sure that there is no disease, infection, swellings or cysts which might be inhibiting your fertility.

With regard to your husband's sperm tests, it is now routine to ask for three repeated tests for the simple reason that one isolated examination can prove to be unreliable. Crudely speaking, therefore, it is now taken to be the best of three, which is a reliable indication of a man's fertility. There is no specific time in any given month at which the seminal fluid sample should be provided, and obviously it was just an accidental inconvenience that on one of the occasions it coincided with your own most fertile time in the month.

Trying for a daughter

Q. I have three boys aged six, four, and two, and we have been trying for a little girl for the past six months. I have been following a timing procedure which is supposed to increase our chances of conceiving a daughter. For the first five months we had intercourse two to three days before ovulation, but as I did not conceive last month, we plucked up courage to go forward by a day or so, and I ovulated about 36 hours later as I had my usual pain at the time. My temperature went up just over two days after intercourse—(the moon was in a 'female' sign at ovulation, too, which is supposed to count for something!), but much to my surprise, my period came 15 days later. As I conceived each of my boys in the first month of trying, we are wondering if my husband is one of those few men who cannot produce female sperms. Why, if sperms and egg were there in the tube, did conception not occur? My temperature stayed up for the full 15 days so I think my hormones are all right. Why do some people have to try for so long? Surely, conception should happen whenever the couple make love at the right time, as long as the man has a good sperm count.
Mrs. O.V., Hants.

A. It would certainly seem from your history that you really do not have any problems over fertility, having conceived so easily in the past, but I warn you that it is not at all uncommon for women to have to wait for between six and 18 months on average for conception and, even though you were fortunate in conceiving very rapidly with your sons, it may well be now that you will have to wait just a little longer.

Whilst it would seem logical that if a man and a woman were to have intercourse at the time of ovulation, there should be no reason why conception should not occur, in practice, nature is fallible in these matters and, just as for some, it can happen the first time, for others, it may often take years for just the right set of circumstances to arise.

It is true that some men carry fewer of the particular chromosomes that result in a female child, but no man is completely incapable of ever having female children.

In answer to your various queries, therefore, I am quite certain it really is only a matter of time before you do conceive. Obviously, statistically, the more babies you have, the greater the chance in the end of having a daughter.

Anxiety effect

Q.   Please help me—two years ago my first baby, a boy, was stillborn. Then five months ago I miscarried at nine weeks. I was so anxious to be pregnant that I was desolate when it ended and I really feel it must have been my anxiety that caused the miscarriage. Could it be that which is stopping me getting pregnant again? I really can't talk to my doctor about it—he seems so rushed, and I think he regards me as a neurotic. At the hospital, too, they process you through their system so quickly you hardly have chance to ask anybody anything. Where could I find someone to explain to me why all this happened? We are reasonably well-off, and my husband feels we should see a London specialist, but how can we go about this?
Mrs. T.L., Surrey.

A.   I can understand how desperate you feel, but there is at least one reassuring thing, which is that you have clearly proved the fertility of both you and your husband.

I don't believe that your failure to conceive at the moment is all psychological—although anxiety and stress can have an influence on the menstrual function. Explain to your family doctor your need for complete reassurance by way of a physical examination and check-up, asking if he could arrange a private appointment with a gynaecologist. Naturally, this facility would be available to you free under the National Health Service, but in certain circumstances, it is worth considering the possibility of some expense to obtain the specialist's individual attention and time.

More than three?

Q.   What is your opinion on large families? I have had three perfectly normal pregnancies and deliveries—my children are now aged four, three, and two, but I want more because I believe that long gaps between children are a bad thing. I've heard it's dangerous to have more than three babies. Is this true?
Mrs. K.C., Lancs.

A.   There is no reason whatsoever why you should not contemplate as many pregnancies as you wish, and there is nothing special about a fourth, fifth or sixth from an obstetric point of view. There is nowadays, no greater risk to foetal or maternal survival, and in view of the fact that your obstetric history has been entirely normal and uncomplicated, there is not the slightest reason to assume that any future confinements would not be exactly like your previous ones. My own opinion is that there is no rule as to how many children it is right to have, as it is purely a question of individual choice.

Further tests

Q.   I am due to see a gynaecologist about my inability to conceive a second child. I have been trying for two years. Our son will be three very shortly, and it took me 14 months to conceive him.

I had been referred to the same gynaecologist I will be seeing soon, and had been told to take my temperature for a few months and if nothing happened he would have had a look at my tubes. My husband had a sperm count but we got no results from this as I became pregnant. Could you tell me if we will probably have to go through the same tests again for secondary infertility, i.e., start with temperatures again, or do you think he'll look at my tubes first?

My husband had to go for a cystoscopy a few months ago and was told he had a lot of inflammation in his prostate, also I was found to have a 'UTI'. Could these have any bearing on our seeming inability to have another baby?

One other point, about two months ago, I caught German measles—does this mean if I do conceive and come into contact with German measles, the baby will be all right?

Mrs. J.C., Notts.

A.   Your gynaecologist will ask you to keep a temperature chart to demonstrate whether you are ovulating or not, and it would probably be helpful if you were to start keeping this straight away so that, when you see him, you will have some evidence to show him with regard to both your menstrual and ovulatory pattern. He will then probably want to do one or two blood tests to assess your hormonal profile, and he may ask your husband to produce samples for sperm counts to be made.

Once he has made a complete physical check of you both, you may find that it is simply a matter of a few months or so of hormone treatment before you become pregnant. Your husband's inflammation in the prostate gland and your 'UTI' (which stands for uninary tract infection) are, I hope, by now resolved. It may be that these minor infections of the genito-urinary system which you have both experienced could have been delaying conception, and with treatment, they will be speedily cleared, so that the fertility of both of you will remain entirely unimpaired.

With regard to your final point, as you have had German measles some two months or so ago, it would now be perfectly safe for you to conceive. You will have developed a natural antibody level to the virus infection of rubella, so you will not be at any risk if you come into contact with the disease, for your natural immunity would protect you and your foetus.

After breast-feeding

Q. I think I must have had a miscarriage, for my period three months ago was very heavy, painful and with clots and lasted for nearly a week. Since then I've only had one scanty period one week early. I've not seen my doctor about it because before that my two periods were scanty and irregular. I only stopped breast-feeding six months ago (my daughter is now a year old and I fed her fully for six months, and then just twice a day for three more). We want another baby, and I have been trying since I stopped breast-feeding. How long does it usually take to become pregnant after breast-feeding? Incidentally, I am on iron prescribed by my doctor because he said it was a good thing for women who breast-feed.
Mrs. C.E., Cheshire.

A. It does seem as if you had a miscarriage, as the character of your menstrual loss seems fairly typical of a pregnancy that was not maintained. To have conceived so early after stopping breast-feeding faced your body with a considerable challenge, and from what you say about your periods, I think that your body was not quite ready yet, and that you are still suffering some degree of hormonal irregularity. Scanty, irregular menstruation is a particular characteristic of this hormonal state.
It often takes three to six months (and sometimes even longer) after pregnancy and a sustained period of breast-feeding, for the body to become ready to conceive again.

Exertion to blame?

Q. I have two little boys, 19 months and seven months. Since my youngest son was born we've been trying for another baby, but so far we've had no luck. I know seven months isn't long but I'd like to know how long to leave it before I go to the doctor. It took us four years to conceive our first baby. I'm 24 and my husband is 28. Is it possible to be three weeks pregnant and have a miscarriage? Since my youngest was born, my periods have been every 30 days, but twice, I was two and three weeks late. I ask this because each time we want to go out I have to take the pram and both children down two flights of steps, and I wondered if this could have caused a miscarriage.

Mrs. B.J., Lincs.

A.   I am sure you need not be unduly concerned, and no gynaecologist would consider beginning any investigations of either you or your husband for at least another 18 months. It is possible that an overdue period could be a miscarriage, but it is often very difficult to tell when a period is only between two and three weeks late. Pregnancy tests are only reliable after a period is more than two weeks overdue, and this is the only way to be sure whether you are pregnant or not. The likelihood of causing a miscarriage by having to lift a pram and children down two flights of steps is remote, for miscarriages are very rarely (if ever) caused by physical effort. When they do occur, it is more often due to hormonal deficiency or some abnormality in the site of implantation in the wall of the uterus.

Moving house

Q.   I am 33 and have a son of 21 months, conceived after trying for only four months, even though we had been married for 10 years. My husband and I have always used the sheath for contraception and for the past three months have been trying for a second baby. I know it is not so easy to conceive a second child, especially after only trying for three months, but I have a slight worry about my periods. They have always been very regular—28 days, but about eight months ago they went irregular (24-26 days interval) and I started losing much more heavily. They have now settled down to 28 days again but I find the first day normal, second day very heavy in which I lose quite a lot of clots (which I didn't have before) and, after the second day, I lose very lightly—it seems as if my period all comes away in one day or so. Can you please explain this change of pattern? Has my body altered in any way?

I would point out that we moved house just before my period pattern changed and had a very worrying time for months before this with the new house, and I wondered if this could have affected me?

Mrs. W.C., Wales.

A.　I am sure you will appreciate that having only been trying to conceive for the last three months or so, there have really been only three occasions on which it might have been possible.

I understand your concern that you may have experienced some physical change in your body because of the change in your menstrual calendar. As your periods have now settled down to a regular pattern, whatever hormonal change may have occurred (very possibly because of the anxiety and disturbances associated with your move), it is now over and it will not in any way have impaired your fertility.

Morning sickness

Q.　I have a son who is nearly two years old, and five months ago I came off the pill to try for a second baby. My periods came regularly every 30 days since I stopped taking the pill, until this month. About a week before my period was due, I started feeling sick, much like the morning sickness I had with my first baby. When my period didn't come on the due date, I convinced myself I was pregnant and I still had the sick feeling at various times of the day. However, 10 days later my period came, and the sickness stopped.

Can one suffer morning sickness before the first period is missed, and could I have been pregnant and lost the baby, or would this just have been a delayed period and the sick feeling due to something else?

Mrs. B.A., Wilts.

A.   You might well have conceived, for it is certainly possible to experience morning sickness as soon as conception occurs—even before the expected period becomes overdue. On the other hand, one also has to recognise that in a state of heightened anxiety about becoming pregnant, sometimes the anxiety itself can cause nausea and an upset feeling generally before an expected period.

Not ready yet

Q.   I had severe toxaemia in my last pregnancy and even now, six months after my baby was born, my blood pressure is not back to normal. My doctor sees me at fortnightly intervals, and I'm on tablets. Could I get pregnant again soon? I do so want another baby.
Mrs. M.R., Cheshire.

A.   It is probably only a matter of time before your blood pressure returns to normal. Toxaemia can place such a severe strain on the kidneys that the blood pressure is high for quite a while afterwards (sometimes for as long as a year to 18 months) and it would be unwise for you to become pregnant again until your blood pressure has returned to normal, and remained so, without treatment, for at least six months.

Post-Caesarean

Q.   How long should I wait after a Caesarean before I get pregnant again? My friend's doctor said it would be three to four years—is he right?
Mrs. M.C., Scotland.

A.   The answer lies in allowing sufficient time for the surgical scar in the womb to heal. One would expect that within three months of the operation, it should be perfectly healed, although most doctors do tend to suggest a period of one year or so before a woman conceives again. Certainly I would have thought that waiting three to four years is erring a little on the side of caution. There is certainly no risk to mother or baby in a conception that takes place earlier—one year later would be the ideal.

Heart problems

Q. I've just had a rather uncomfortable forceps delivery of my first baby—I had to have forceps because I have a heart valve murmur. What I would like to know is will any future deliveries be as uncomfortable, and will I always have to have forceps? Secondly, what is the best age to have a second baby—I'm 29 and a bit worried about getting too old. Lastly, what is the minimum time I should wait before I become pregnant again?
Mrs. W.D., Leics.

A. Second and subsequent deliveries are always very much easier than the first, and whilst an epidural anaesthetic may be suggested because of your cardiac weakness, you will find that in view of the increased size of the birth passages and the greater effectiveness of the muscles concerned, you will probably be able to give birth without the assistance of forceps.
As to how long to wait before starting a second baby, this can only be a matter of opinion; personally, I would suggest that when your child is three or four, out of nappies, and getting ready for school, would be the most convenient time for you to conceive again. Because you are 29, it might be sensible to try to conceive a little earlier since it may take as long as a year. As to a minimum time that you should wait, in view of your experience last time, it will probably be best to wait at least another year or 18 months before becoming pregnant again, to allow all the tissues to heal, your menstruation to return to its regular pattern, and for you to be able to handle all the work associated with two small children.

Never too old

Q. My son was born a year ago, and afterwards I was very depressed, tearful and bad-tempered. I don't know why; I so dearly wanted a baby and I feel I'm to blame for not being a perfect mother. I'm much better now though, and I feel I've passed through a tunnel and come out the other end. I'm 33 now and would dearly love another baby but am I too old? I've heard all sorts of stories about the risks older mothers run and the things that go wrong. What do you think?
Mrs. M.E., Staffs.

A. It is obvious that you suffered from acute post-natal depression. It can happen to anyone, and it was certainly not your fault.
At 33, you are certainly not too old to conceive. In fact, you still have 13 or 14 reproductive years ahead of you when you can have as large a family as you want. There is no need to be unduly concerned about the possibility of anything happening to you or the baby because of your age.

A cloud

Q. We have a lovely baby boy of three, but since then I've had another pregnancy that ended in a stillbirth. As a result, I've had severe depression, and my doctor has prescribed tablets for me. I keep feeling that perhaps I'm not a natural mother, and as I'm approaching 35, I'm too old anyway. I'm insecure and would like to know whether I should get pregnant again. I'd like a rest for a few months before facing it—but how long should I wait?
Mrs. H.J., Sussex.

A. A stillbirth is a most tragic experience. This sort of experience can be much more painful for the more mature woman who might feel that her reproductive years are slipping past, and your depressive reaction to this, was, I feel, entirely understandable.
My advice, however, is to look forward confidently to

the future, knowing that you have at least demonstrated the fertility of you and your husband. The birth of your son three years ago also demonstrates that your body is capable of carrying a pregnancy through to term and delivering a normal, healthy baby.

If you allow your body some six to nine months or so of rest from the challenge of pregnancy, you may find that you could contemplate another pregnancy. By then your quite natural depression will probably have lifted and you will no longer need to take medication. You will receive, because of your obstetric history, the most scrupulous care and specialist attention, throughout your antenatal period.

CHAPTER VI

The Older Mother

Too old?

Q. Friends have been telling me that after the age of 30, it is very difficult to start having babies. I'm 31 and now I'm worried in case we've left it too late. What is the latest age at which a woman can have her first baby? Both my husband and I are perfectly healthy, and my periods are regular.
Mrs. S.N., Midlands.

A. There are literally thousands of women who have their first babies in their early and middle forties, and there is no reason whatsoever for you to believe what people have been telling you. Naturally a woman's fertility in her mid-thirties is not quite as high as it was in her mid-twenties, but it has not deteriorated all that much.
The age at which a woman can have her first baby depends, quite naturally, on the duration of her reproductive life, but the latest age ever reported in medical literature was a woman of 52. That should not be taken as a guide, merely as an example! You should have every encouragement to plan your first baby at whatever age you wish. It might take you just a little bit longer to conceive than it might a younger woman, but there is no reason at all why you should not be successful.

Is it the menopause?

Q. I am 31, with a three-year-old son. My husband and I are desperate for another child but have had no success for the past 18 months. I am so afraid I have started the menopause. For the past three months my periods have been accompanied by hot sweats, mainly in the night, but also some in the day. Prior to this two things happened which could have upset my system:— I went on the pill for three months in the hope I might become pregnant afterwards. I have never used the pill before. At exactly the same time, a dear relative of my age contracted leukaemia. I was under great stress visiting her and watching her die. The hot sweats began just before the funeral. I have only heard of hot flushes as associated with the menopause, and I feel utterly heartbroken that it could begin at my age.
My husband feels there must be another reason though I do not agree. At the moment I feel I cannot face my doctor with all this as I don't think he would take me seriously.
Mrs. D.S., Devon.

A. It is extremely unlikely from what you tell me that the menopause is responsible for your symptoms. There are many conditions which cause night sweats, and two of the commonest are anxiety and glandular fever. The latter can very easily be diagnosed by a blood test, and you should ask your doctor to do a routine blood test on you to check, firstly, whether you are anaemic and, secondly, whether there is a possibility of your having caught this kind of virus infection.
Worry and anxiety are also a common cause of this condition, but tend to be associated at the same time with palpitations of the heart, some shaking or tremor of the limbs, along with a dry mouth, and this, too, can be treated if your doctor confirms the diagnosis. Indeed, I would think that in view of the sad loss of your relative from leukaemia, it is not at all unlikely that this might well be the cause of your present symptoms.
With regard to your fertility, I am sure you will appreciate, too, that anxiety often diminishes fertility, sometimes even by suppressing ovulation, but you can look forward

with confidence to full recovery in due course. I am quite certain that, in time, you will become pregnant again.

"Senile" at 40

Q. I'm 39 and had my fourth baby (normal delivery, eight-pound son) three years ago, but my doctor said when I told him I'd like a fifth that I was getting senile! Naturally I'm very worried about the possibility of having a handicapped baby—but I've heard there are tests for this. What are they, and are they dangerous? Also, are there a lot of problems in labour for the older woman?
Mrs. S.R., Israel.

A. At 39, you are certainly not senile, and particularly in view of the fact that you had a baby perfectly normally three years ago, you are obviously in the peak of reproductive condition. I do understand, however, that you are naturally concerned about the possibility of giving birth to a handicapped baby. Tests for Down's syndrome (mongolism) and also spina bifida, along with several other foetal abnormalities, can be conducted on a woman of mature years any time up to the 20th week of her pregnancy. They are undertaken firstly by means of an ultrasound scan to determine the exact position of the placenta and the foetus and then by the introduction of a very tiny needle through the anaesthetised wall of the abdomen in order to draw off some of the fluid that surrounds the foetus. This test, known as the amniocentesis test, is then used to assess whether there is any foetal abnormality. There are no risks to either mother or baby when the test is properly conducted by experienced people—and this form of surveillance is now becoming much more widely available.

As to whether the older mother has any difficulties during pregnancy or labour that the younger mother does not, it always depends on the individual. Having delivered your son three years ago without any difficulty, you will obviously not have the slightest problem with any further pregnancies, for quite obviously your muscular tissues and genital organs are in excellent condition. It is usually only the mature mother who has not had a baby for many years who experiences difficulties.

Age problems?

Q.   Why does an older woman find it more difficult to get pregnant?

A.   The idea that fertility decreases with a woman's age is based on the evidence that a woman conceives much more easily in her early twenties than she does in her early thirties, and often only with some difficulty in her early forties. The reasons are numerous. They vary from a depression in the fertility of her husband to ageing of the fallopian tubes, the ovaries and a reduction in the frequency of ovulation, as well as an impairment of the internal uterine environment. In the older woman, particularly one in her forties, for example, a change in the uterine tissue takes place leading to fibroids (fibrous replacements of normal tissue), and this can impair the prospects of implantation, even after conception has taken place.

Life begins at . . .?

Q.   I'm about to get married for the first time—at the age of 40. I do want a baby and would welcome your advice on how long we should wait to see if I'm fertile or not. Is it only a faint hope?
Mrs. D.G., Scotland.

A.   Certainly there is no medical reason whatsoever why you should not have a baby. You do not tell me whether your menstruation is regular or not, but I would assume that it must be so or you would have mentioned it.
I suggest that you keep an ovulation chart, recording your temperature daily and looking out for the dip and subsequent rise in your morning temperature that usually occurs somewhere round the 10th to 14th day

after a period has started. If you are able to identify this as being your most fertile period over a time interval of three to four months or so, it will help you and your husband to take advantage of this peak in fertility. If, however, there is no clear evidence of ovulation, I feel you should ask your doctor to refer you to a gynaecologist for investigations.

There are many forms of medical treatment available nowadays to stimulate ovulation, and if your husband is fertile and your ovulation is chemically stimulated, the possibility of your conceiving will obviously be enhanced. There are literally many thousands of women each year who conceive not only in their early forties but many of them in their mid and occasionally late forties, too, so you could have confidence in the possibility that it may well occur for you as well.

Why more daughters?

Q. We've three children, all sons, and the youngest is 10—but we'd love a daughter. We're both 43 now and feel time is running out, but I've read that in the over forties there is a much greater chance of having a baby girl. Why is this? Are these statistics reliable?
Mrs. L. D., Beds.

A. You have every reason to be confident that both you and your husband are fertile, and although, quite naturally, you feel that approaching the age of 43, time is running out, I can reassure you that births are reported every year to women in their late forties and, last year in America, there were two recorded cases of perfectly normal healthy babies being delivered to women who were aged 52.

The statistics concerning the greater incidence of girls, rather than boys, being born to women over 40 are interesting and true. The reason for this is not clear, but there is little doubt that it is somehow related to the fact that more first babies born to younger mothers are male than female. However, you still might have a son the next time, despite the fact that the statistical trend would seem to suggest the opposite possibility.

Settle for one?

Q.   Please could you help me to make up my mind? I was pregnant for the first time when I was 34, but at six and a half months, I miscarried identical twin boys. I was so ill from the third month until I lost the babies that it just put me off trying again, but in the back of my mind I was longing for a baby, and I knew my husband wanted children as much as I did. Last year, four years later, I gave birth to a lovely baby girl after a normal pregnancy and labour. She is now 13 months old. I am 40 this month and would very much like another baby. Do you think we should take the chance or be content with the precious daughter we have? Mrs. S.F., Lancs.

A.   It is obvious that having given birth last year to a perfectly normal and healthy baby girl, there is no reason why you should not have another healthy child. The fact that some years ago you suffered a miscarriage is not likely to influence the immediate future, for it is common to miscarry with multiple pregnancies.
Your age means that you should not leave it for too long. If you feel you want to increase your family, there is no medical reason whatsoever why you should not do so.

Twins again?

Q.   I will be 44 in June, and both my husband and I would dearly love to have another baby. I have five children aged 21, 18, 13 and 10-year-old non-identical twins. I do have a fantastic relationship with all my children, and motherhood has been the greatest experience in my life with not too many problems. If I were to become pregnant again what are the chances of me having twins again? Mrs. W.I., Bucks.

A.   It is never too late to start again. The chances of a multiple pregnancy are, however, definitely reduced with ageing, since non-identical twins or more depend on multiple ovulation occurring. Since ovulation frequently diminishes with age, the likelihood of this happening is lessened. Identical twins can still occur, however, but these are the rarest kind.

One of her own

Q. I've just got married again at 44 after being widowed two years ago. We had no children of our own, but I've fostered lots of them. (My first husband couldn't have children, although after all the tests I was told I was all right.) What are the real facts about having a baby at my age? I feel so indecisive about it all —my periods are regular still, and I dearly love children. I still keep in touch with all of those we used to call 'our family', and they all come to see me just as if I had been their real mother.
Mrs. R.G., Isle of Wight.

A. I do understand your dilemma about starting a family at the age of 44. It may be medically true to state that no woman, provided she is still ovulating, is ever too old to have a baby, but there are a great number of things to be taken into account when the decision to start a family at this age is taken. Firstly, it is not necessarily quite so easy to conceive; secondly, there is a greater likelihood of complications with regard to the continuation of the pregnancy; and thirdly there are more possibilities of the child being affected by some form of genetic handicap. However, it is obvious that you have a great deal of love and affection for children. Why not go ahead and let nature decide for you?

Success for some . . .

Q. I am 48 and have just had my fifth baby—a lovely daughter. My eldest daughter—a nurse—is now married and I am actually a grandmother as well! The two sons are at university and my next daughter is about to leave school and go to secretarial college. I went through all sorts of worries about this last 'mistake' of ours but the doctors were very good and I had all the tests—in the end I delivered her myself. The paediatrician said she's as normal and as bright as all the others.

A.   It is particularly nice to hear that you have a new baby and you have no reason to believe that there is any concern about the possibility of mental handicap. The risks are always slightly greater for a woman of your age, but, in fact, you have demonstrated clearly that your fertility is unimpaired, your uterus is perfectly capable of carrying through a normal pregnancy to full-term, and that your baby was entirely unaffected, despite your age.

Unlikely

Q.   I shall be 51 soon and only started the menopause last year. In the past, my husband used a sheath, but in later years we have used the 'safe period'. Last year, I missed a period or so, and this year I missed three on the run. I don't know whether I'm still fertile or not. Is it possible to become pregnant at 51?
Mrs. H.M., Suffolk.

A.   It is always a problem when a woman reaches the menopause, and there is uncertainty with regard to fertility. Once you have passed a year without menstruation you can assume that you will not be able to conceive.
It is possible to become pregnant at 51, if a woman is still ovulating and menstruating regularly, although it is very rare. In your case, I would feel that your reproductive time is coming to a close, and you will probably find the gap between your menstrual periods continues to lengthen.

CHAPTER VII

Genetic Problems

Sperm worry

Q. Earlier this year my three-year-old son had skull X-rays taken following slight concussion. My husband was asked to stand with him whilst he was being X-rayed. However, my son was rather frightened by everything, and my husband had to stand close to him and help to hold him still. I was called in after it appeared he had moved and further X-rays were taken (five in all, we think) with me standing behind some sort of screen holding him at one end and my husband at the other end of the screen.

I am now 17 weeks pregnant although I was not pregnant at the time my son was X-rayed. I am certain that I conceived one week later and am worried that the sperm which fertilised the egg may have been affected by the X-rays. We did not have intercourse between the day of the X-rays and the time of conception, so that the sperm were 'there' at the time my son was X-rayed with my husband standing very close to him. I understand that it is not recommended that a woman is X-rayed in the early stages of pregnancy, but what about a man? Mrs. M.J., Yorks.

A. Any spermatozoa that might, by some remote possibility, have been damaged by exposure to X-rays, would not be capable of fertilising an egg cell. Only normal undamaged cells would achieve this. Secondly, the intensity of X-rays used to take a picture of the skull in a young child would be very low indeed and not scattered over a wide area, so that even though your husband was standing close to your son, it is most unlikely that his genital area was exposed to irradiation. Furthermore, from what you tell me, it does seem that both you and your husband stood behind a protective screen, and as these are made of lead, they provide perfect protection from X-rays.

A serious illness

Q. I had a melanoma removed from my right leg 10 years ago, just above my ankle, with quite a large area of flesh taken away. Four years later there was a blockage in the lymph gland of the same leg and that was removed. Three years later a tiny lump was removed from my back which was also slightly affected.

My husband and I would very much like to have children, and when, before I got married three years ago, I asked the specialist in charge of my case about having having a family, he didn't feel there would be any problem. After having the last lump removed two years ago, however, we were advised to wait for two years before starting a family.

I became pregnant last year—the coil I had fitted before I got married should have been changed after two years, but I was not informed of this and, as the coil had 'expired' it was no longer effective as a means of contraception. I went to see the specialist when the pregnancy was confirmed, and he strongly advised me not to go through with the pregnancy since he felt it might trigger off my old problem. The most distressing point was that he felt it wiser to give up the idea of producing children altogether. I had a termination at two months. My husband and I have complete faith in the specialist and felt the choice wasn't ours since we respected his advice. We had weeks and weeks of depression and disappointment and were rather bewildered as to why at one point I was told that it would be all right to have children and have now been advised not to consider it. The specialist said: 'It is not dangerous enough to say definitely not, but dangerous enough to say possibly not'. After a great deal of thought, my husband and I decided we would apply to become adoptive parents. The specialists and my doctors are in full support of this idea, so we went ahead and wrote to the agencies which cater for our area and with which we qualified to apply. We wrote to six altogether and were most disappointed to be told by them all that their lists were closed and would not open in the forseeable future. My husband is a self-employed farmer and I am a school teacher. We are church people—I teach in Sunday school and am on the Parochial Church Council, but unfortunately, the Church of England Adoption Society have an age limit of 40 for the husband and my husband is 42. I am 34.

We would be most grateful for any advice or suggestions you could give on the subject of the melanoma in relation to pregnancy and about adoption.
Mrs. B.G., Scotland.

A.   One of the problems with recurrent conditions associated with cell growth is that in pregnancy there is a considerable acceleration in all forms of cell growth, and quite obviously your specialist was concerned about the possibility of recurrence of the melanoma, and despite the upset over your termination, I am quite sure that you were given the best advice.

Now that you have made the decision to adopt, you are running into a very common problem. There is such a shortage of babies for adoption that the possibilities of adopting for prospective couples are getting fewer and fewer. Because of the shortage of babies, most of the Adoption Societies now make many restrictive rules with regard to prospective parents, but I wonder whether, because of your connection with the Church of England, you might not try and prevail on The Church of England Adoption Society to accept you and your husband as prospective parents in view of the fact that your husband's age is only just over the limit. If you can assemble on your behalf some 'official' recommendations from friends and colleagues in authority in the church locally, that could be forwarded on your behalf, they might perhaps then bend their rules just a little in your favour.

Blood group problems

Q. My blood group is O Rhesus negative and my husband's is O Rhesus positive. I had a baby last year who is Rhesus positive. At the antenatal classes I was advised that I would need an anti-D injection within 24 hours of the birth if my baby was Rhesus positive. I asked the staff a couple of times after the birth whether I would require an injection and was told that since I hadn't had one, I obviously didn't require one. I naturally assumed that my baby's blood group was the same as mine. However, 75 hours after the birth I was given the injection since he was found to be Rhesus positive. I tried to find out while I was in hospital whether the fact that I was given the injection after a long period would affect any future pregnancies but my query was brushed aside and I was told to think about the baby I had got and not about any future children.
I have once again begun to worry about the effect this may have on any future pregnancies. Please could you advise me on this? Also, although we would very much like another child, I don't think I could take the chance of it being affected in any way because of the blood incompatibility, so would it be better if I didn't have any more children?
Mrs. B.J., Surrey.

A. It was surprising to learn that there was some delay in your being given the anti-D injection. It was, I think, most remiss of your medical advisers not to administer it to you as soon as possible after your baby was delivered, and his blood group was identified.
Nevertheless, the injection will certainly have suppressed very largely any antibody response to the release of Rhesus positive antigens from the placental site in your uterus. It is most likely that if you were to have a blood test now to determine whether there were any Rhesus positive antibodies in your system, it would prove to be

negative, and this is certainly a way in which you could have your mind set at rest, if your doctor felt prepared to arrange this for you.

Similarly, should you conceive again, you will of course have the standard antibody test undertaken as soon as your pregnancy is confirmed, and the tests will be continued at periodic intervals throughout the pregnancy to ascertain whether any antibody rise occurs as your pregnancy continues. If you do want to have any more children, therefore, there is no reason why you should not go ahead.

Incompatability

Q. I am 28 this year, and when I had my daughter three years ago, it was discovered that we had AB/O incompatibility and she became very jaundiced, her level of bilrubin reached $17\frac{1}{2}$ and I was told that if it went up to 18, the doctor would then do an exchange transfusion. She also had an umbilical infection which required treatment. Happily, at 11 days, she was discharged and is now absolutely fine.

I would love to have another baby and on consulting a geneticist was told that another baby would have a 50/50 chance of the same trouble and if it were affected, labour would probably be induced at 36 weeks —I gather because the blood mingles more in the last month. The geneticist also said that because of the baby's immaturity the lungs would not be properly developed and, therefore, there was a slight risk of brain damage.

Could you give me your opinion on the problems of immaturity and whether you think it would be wise for me to have another baby?

Mrs. P.M., Devon.

A. The condition of AB/O incompatibility is well recognised, even though it is not particularly common, and it is a consequence of the incompatibility between your husband's blood group and your own. When you are pregnant with a baby of a 'foreign' blood group to your own, you develop antibodies which are passed back to the baby through the placenta which then start to damage the developing baby's blood cells. The geneticist's advice is correct in that you would have a 50-50 chance of the same trouble occurring, but not quite correct in his explaining how such a pregnancy would be handled. Indeed, if there were signs of a high level of antibodies in your blood stream, premature labour would be induced, but if the signs were not present, then the pregnancy would be allowed to go to full term. With a 50-50 chance, therefore, of everything being perfectly normal, I think you are in a reasonable position to decide whether you want to increase your family or not. There are many women who, with much slimmer chances of a normal pregnancy, have, nevertheless, had perfectly normal deliveries of healthy babies.

Blindness

Q. My mother-in-law is 56 and has been going blind for some years. We have now discovered that she has retinitis pigmentosa. She is the only member of her large family to have the disease or to have ever shown any signs of it, although I know it is hereditary. Should we have our two-year-old daughter screened for the disease now? If so, where? What are her chances of developing it? Should we have genetic counselling before thinking of having another child? I suddenly feel very worried about my daughter's future and have a sense of guilt that she may become blind in turn, too. Mrs. L.P., Middlesex.

A. This really is a most distressing and incurable condition, but I can reassure you that it is not necessarily genetically dominant. Indeed, the fact that no other members of the family have shown any signs of this disorder is evidence of this, but in the interest of complete reassurance, you should perhaps ask your family doctor to arrange for an ophthalmic specialist's opinion on your husband and your daughter, just in case, and at the same time, for advice from a genetic counsellor. Retinitis pigmentosa is a condition which may only develop in later years, and whilst it would be exceptionally difficult for an ophthalmic specialist to detect any changes in a two-year-old child, the evidence of a full optical assessment of your husband would be most reassuring from the point of view of your own family, and the advice of a genetic counsellor as to whether there is any particular sex link with just the female side of the family would be helpful and reassuring.

It would be a most sensible step for you to take before conceiving again.

Muscular dystrophy

Q. We've recently married, and although we're a 'mature' couple (I'm 32 and my husband is 45), we'd like to have children. There is one serious problem—in my husband's family, there is a history of muscular dystrophy. (His brother's family doctor said it was 'Duchenne-type'). Could my husband be carrying this gene since I understand it is a congenital abnormality and would any children I conceive suffer from it? If so, what tests could I have and how could I find out, after I conceive, if the baby is affected?
Mrs. F.P., Merseyside.

A. The type of muscular dystrophy you describe is carried only by the male line and is suffered only by male children. As a result of this knowledge, its incidence is gradually diminishing, for where there is a family history of this condition, a woman can be offered a scanning test and amniocentesis before she is 20 weeks pregnant, which will determine the sex of the child. At the same time, in larger teaching hospital areas, tests can be done on the foetal fluids to see whether the particular genetic pattern is present or not. If this is so, then a termination of the pregnancy can be offered. With regard to your husband carrying the recessive gene, this is at present thought to be impossible with the Duchenne type of muscular dystrophy.

My advice has to be something of a generalisation, and much more specific advice could be obtained from a genetic counsellor. Should you contemplate increasing your family in the future, you might ask your general practitioner if he could refer you for this kind of help, when I am sure you would be given much more specific guidance.

Colour vision defects

Q.   I have a little boy who is 18 months old and I've just learnt that there is colour-blindness in my husband's family. My husband is not affected but could my son be? Both his older nephews on my husband's side are. How and when could my son be tested?
Mrs. R.E., London.

A.   There are, in fact, several different types of colour blindness, the commonest being the red/green, whose victims see both those colours as grey. This does tend to be genetically linked and predominantly a male defect, so there is, I am afraid, quite a strong possibility that your little boy might have inherited this disadvantage in view of your family history. It is, however, not a very serious problem, and many people reach adulthood before they know that they are colour blind, particularly if the defect is only minor. It is possible for tests to be undertaken on young children to detect this condition, but usually it is necessary to wait until they are talking and able to follow simple instructions (around two to three). You must mention it to any doctors performing child assessment tests on your little boy, but if he should prove in the end to be colour blind, I would certainly not regard this as a severe handicap.

Heart defects

Q.   My sister has just lost her second baby—stillborn due to a congenital heart defect. The same thing happened to her two years ago, another stillborn boy with heart defects. Could this be genetic? How could she find out and will any future babies she has be affected?
Mrs. D.F., Beds.

A.   The occurrence of congenital malformation of the heart is well recognised, but the incidence is around one in 10,000 cases. For your sister to have had two successive children with a defect incompatible with life is indeed far more than would normally be expected statistically.

Without knowing precisely what the malformation was, I cannot offer you any clear explanation, but I can suggest some practical steps for your sister to take once she has recovered from her tragic experience. She should ask her family doctor for a full explanation with regard to the post-mortem findings on the two babies. Once she has these, she should ask for referral to a specialist in genetic counselling who will be able to take the matter much further and see whether there is in fact any dominant genetic defect which your sister or her husband may be carrying. If there is she should obviously not have any further children. If not then, although she would obviously be worried, she could at least be sure that the statistical likelihood of a third child being affected would be exceptionally remote.

Vaccination advice

Q.   How long should a woman wait after a German measles vaccination before she can conceive and be sure that the baby will not be genetically damaged, or that she will not get the disease herself?
Mrs. R.S., Leics.

A.   At least two months should be allowed to elapse before conception, and preferably three. The reason for this is that the vaccination consists of the live virus, which can remain in the body for some three to four weeks after administration. The body does not develop the antibodies that are necessary to prevent the person from ever contracting this disease again until some eight weeks have passed after the vaccine is administered. The vaccination cannot in any way lead to genetic damage in the baby conceived if the time lapse of two, or preferably three, months is observed.

Two years to wait

Q. I'm just getting over jaundice, and I have been told by my doctor that I must not get pregnant for two years at least. Is this correct? Why is this rule laid down? What would happen if I did get pregnant before the two years were up?
Mrs. R.G., Hants.

A. Jaundice, or hepatitis, as the disease is called, is very distressing and upsetting. It is a disease of the liver, caused by a virus, and can cause a great deal of liver damage. It can take up to two years or so for the liver cells to repair themselves after this infection. Indeed, in many patients who have various blood tests to assess liver function, the results are still not normal for as long as a year to 18 months after all the jaundice and yellowness in the skin have cleared.
The advice that you were given was sensible, since pregnancy can make a great deal of extra work for the liver. Should you accidentally get pregnant, you may find that although your baby is perfectly well, you may suffer a return of your original symptoms, and this is why the delay has been suggested.

Sex determination

Q. How can I make sure I conceive a boy—or if we want one later, a girl? I've read about lots of ways of ensuring that either only boys are conceived, or only girls. Is there a safe way of doing this?
Mrs. S.M., Midlands.

A. There are no reliable methods for choosing the sex of a child. A great deal of publicity has surrounded this subject with regard to the use of temperature charts, vaginal douches, special creams and even the timing of intercourse at a particular part of the menstrual calendar, but in the final statistical analysis none of these methods have any influence whatsoever on the sex of the child. Any method will certainly have a 50 per cent chance of being right, since there are only two sexes!

Therefore, many of the myths continue to be propagated in various articles and stories, and I am sorry to have to tell you that scientifically there is no truth in them whatsoever.

CHAPTER VIII

Special Problems

Must not become pregnant

Q.   I am an agoraphobic, and at times my nerves are really bad. My doctor has prescribed Nardil and Librium tablets.
I would dearly love another child, but I realise that at the moment, with my nerves as they are, it is out of the question. My doctor has told me to take precautions but should I conceive, would the growing baby be harmed by my medicines?
Mrs. A.M., Kent.

A.   Nardil is an antidepressant that works by inhibiting a particular enzyme in the brain called monoamine oxidase, and works by overcoming the excessive production of this enzyme, which is thought to cause depression when it is present in excess. Certainly Nardil would affect the growing baby, and it is most important not to become pregnant whilst you are taking it. For that reason you should make sure that your contraceptive precautions are completely reliable. If they are not, you should consult your Family Planning Clinic in order to obtain the most effective advice, or ask your family doctor to make arrangements for you. If you do not find that the treatment has brought about a considerable improvement in your symptoms and your feelings within the next three months, then you should ask your doctor to refer you to a psychiatrist in order to obtain the most skilled help possible. Nowadays many psychiatrists find that forms of psychotherapy and group therapy are as helpful in treating your condition as drug treatment, if not more so in some cases.

A question of priorities

Q. I have been treated for depression for many years, and for the last two I have been prescribed Ativan tablets, which I take four times a day. I'm a very anxious person and even the simplest things can upset me. I would like to have a baby though—could I have one and still take the tablets?
Mrs. H.M., Avon.

A. Ideally conception should not occur while anti-depressant tablets such as Ativan are being taken.
You should concentrate on gradually weaning yourself off Ativan and, provided you can achieve this and remain happily adjusted, there is no reason why you should not contemplate conceiving. If you were to become pregnant, however, while taking this drug, you would spend many months worrying about the possibility of foetal abnormality and, in fact, the manufacturers do specifically state that Ativan should not be taken by women in the early weeks of pregnancy. In your case the first priority is your full and satisfactory recovery from your psychological disorder. If you can achieve this in the not too distant future, having a baby can become your first priority.

Long-standing problem

Q. Please tell me what causes a cervical erosion and polyps. I've had this trouble for years now and I can't understand why I don't seem to get better. I've just seen the gynaecologist now for the fifth time, and at last he has cauterised me and done a D & C—having tried out all sorts of creams and pessaries. My period hasn't come

yet, though—will I be cured now and could I start a baby?
Mrs. D.H., Wales.

A.   You are unfortunate in having had both a cervical erosion and later a cervical polyp.
Basically, an erosion of the cervix is like a chronic soreness on any part of the skin where the normal surface cells are worn away by minor but chronic infection, and the whole area continues to weep and ooze fluid as it tries to repair itself. Very often it does not succeed and has to be cauterised in order to clean up the area and give it a good chance to heal. However, sometimes certain cells in the damaged area overgrow a little and form polyps, which are rather like little skin tags. These can leak fluid, sometimes blood-stained, and have to be removed surgically. Before treatment, they often cause chronic discomfort and irritation. However, it would seem that you are well on the way towards recovery now, and once your periods return to normal, there is no reason why you should not start a baby.

Cone biopsy

Q.   I had to have a cone biopsy last year, and the result of this was satisfactory. My husband and I want another baby very much and, in fact, we had hoped to have had one before now, but of course we had to postpone it because of the biopsy. The surgeon told me that I can have one whenever we like. I am extremely upset, however, after reading an article by a midwife in which she says that conception and birth after this operation can be difficult. How much more difficult is it likely to be to conceive? I conceived easily with my two sons aged eight and five. I am now 32, and I know that fertility gradually diminishes from the age of about 30 (my periods are very regular). How does the biopsy make it more difficult and what complications can it cause during the birth? Also how long should we try before seeking further advice?
Mrs. W.K., Dorset.

A.   I can reassure you with complete confidence that the standard cone biopsy, which only removes a tiny amount of material from the cervical canal, has no effect whatsoever on subsequent fertility, conception, pregnancy or the conduct of labour. There are considerable variations in the amount of tissue removed from the cervix, and the article that you read must have been referring to one where a large portion of the cervix had been taken away. In view of the fact that yours was simply a routine cone biopsy, the suggestions do not in any way apply to you. You will find, therefore, that your opportunities for conception are not impaired, and you can go ahead and try for a baby. If, after nine months to a year or so of trying, you have not become pregnant, you should ask your family doctor to arrange for the usual fertility investigations.

A serious danger

Q.   I had a baby five years ago and had a pulmonary embolism on the second post-natal day. I have never understood why this happened, though I know clotting in the blood does tend to occur after childbirth. Could you explain why? I was told never to have another baby, and my husband has had a vasectomy.
Mrs. W.M., Midlands.

A.   Pulmonary embolism is a rather rare condition but all women are prone to the occurrence of thrombosis during the immediate post-natal period. Whilst thrombosis used to be more common years ago, particularly in the legs, because women were kept far too long in bed after their confinement without exercise, nevertheless it still occurs from time to time in other parts of the body, and there is often no way of predicting in whom it will occur or when. The reason that women are prone to it in the post-natal period is twofold. Firstly, towards the end of pregnancy, the blood returns sluggishly from the lower limbs to the heart, because of the size of the pregnant uterus. In other words there is mechanical obstruction. Secondly, after delivery the oestrogen level rises, and this predisposes the blood to more rapid clotting. This effect is desirable from nature's point of view in order to reduce the possibility of post-natal haemorrhage, but if it becomes excessive, it is liable to provoke unwanted clotting.

Fear of asthma attack

Q. I have had very bad asthma since I was a child, and as I've just got married, I dread the thoughts of becoming pregnant and either losing my baby during an attack of asthma or dying in labour because of it. Is this likely to happen?
Mrs. B.P., Lincs.

A. You are bound to be anxious and worried about the possibility of getting an attack of asthma during pregnancy or labour, but this is most unlikely to happen. During pregnancy many of the hormones which normally circulate throughout the body are considerably increased and one in particular, known as cortisone, circulates in especially high levels. The treatment for asthma is cortisone, for this overcomes the spasm effect that occurs in the respiratory passages when asthma is present. You can see, therefore, that the body, in fact, protects the mother by producing naturally a substance which, in the non-pregnant state, has to be given as medical treatment. Even women who suffer chronic asthma, having to take many different forms of medication to control their respiratory difficulties, find that they are in the best of health whenever they are pregnant.

The cause of pain

Q. Please can you help me with my problem over the pains I get in my abdomen? One is almost constant in my right side, low down. I've seen several doctors about it, but they have always said it is not due to my internal organs. It comes and goes but sometimes lasts for hours and is not associated with my periods in any way. The second problem I've had ever since my last baby and it is in the front of my pelvis. When I had my daughter, I heard a cracking sound at the front as she was delivered and it has given me agony ever since. If I bend down, open my legs wide (or even when I'm sitting on the toilet) I get this terrible sharp pain just underneath my pubic hair and above my vagina. What could it be? I dread having another baby in case it makes it worse.

Mrs. R.W., Lancs.

A.   There are two possibilities with regard to the cause of your pains. One is that you have a small ovarian cyst, but it would be strange if it had not been diagnosed by the various doctors who have examined you in the past. Therefore, the second most likely cause, the 'grumbling appendix', is probably involved. In similar cases, quite often a chronically inflamed appendix is found, and has to be removed.

Having said that, however, very frequently these conditions, called 'the grumbling appendix', do in fact disappear without treatment, and it could easily be that the attacks of pain become less and less frequent and gradually disappear altogether. Next time you get the pain for any length of time you should ask your doctor to examine you so that a diagnosis can be made.

The second condition is caused by the female sex hormones that circulate throughout the body in pregnancy and cause nearly all joints to become lax and loose. Some women seem particularly prone to suffering the effect of this looseness in a rather painful way on the frontal pelvic joint. This joint, which is in the middle of the pubic hairline, is normally rigid. However, in order to allow some degree of expansion of the pelvis when a woman is pregnant the joint loosens slightly and sometimes widens a little, but in most cases the joint re-tightens after giving birth. You obviously went through the loosening, probably with some straining of this joint, and it has not as yet completely tightened up. You should ask your doctor to refer you to an orthopaedic specialist, for in certain circumstances, long-acting anaesthetic injections can be made into the joint area which immediately relieve all the pain. Should it not be corrected, it will certainly be aggravated by any further pregnancies and could easily, in fact, get worse.

Ovarian pain

Q. I have been married for five years, and my husband and I have a happy loving relationship, but each time we have intercourse I have a pain on the right side of my body, just below waist level. It started quite mildly soon after we were married, but I ignored it thinking that it would disappear after having a baby. However, I have not had a baby yet, and the pain has become much worse even with very gentle love-making. Deeper penetration has now become impossible as this not only causes pain in my side but also sends a cramp-like feeling down my right leg. I am sure that I would enjoy sex much more if it wasn't for this problem. My periods are quite normal and painless.
My general health is good and I don't have a weight problem—but I do want a baby soon. The pain doesn't occur except on intercourse—what could be the cause? Mrs. K.L., Bucks.

A. The pain you describe sounds like ovarian pain, and the probably cause is either a slight prolapse of the ovary so that it is lying closer to the top of the vagina than normal, or some very minor abnormality such as a small cyst on the right ovary. It is extremely uncomfortable to have pressure put on the ovary and, in the circumstances, I am sure that you should ask your doctor to refer you to a gynaecologist for a full and complete internal investigation. This will involve a very small tube being inserted through a tiny incision in your abdominal wall, under a local anaesthetic, so the ovary can be inspected from inside by means of the light which illuminates the area at the end of the tube. If there is any cyst on the ovary it will be dealt with and your fertility improved.

It always hurts

Q. We've been married a year now (I'm 19), but I have a problem that I'm very embarrassed about—my vagina's too dry for sex. My husband is understanding, but it always hurts me whenever he starts to make love to me. I'm sure I'll never have a baby because of this—

it even hurts me to try tampons and I gave up because I got sore when I went on trying them. Is there anything I can do? Do you think there is something wrong with me? Mrs. B.J., Cheshire.

A.   There are two causes of this problem, and one of them is the vaginal infection called thrush. This is by no means a serious infection, but is a great nuisance and can, in certain cases, make the vagina dry and sore. Your doctor will prescribe some cream and pessaries for you to insert in your vagina each night which will rapidly solve the problem. One of the signs of thrush is often vaginal soreness (also irritation and itching around the outside of the vagina), and certainly if you find yourself developing any of these signs, you should see your doctor.

The second cause is very much more simple. Sometimes, insufficient lubrication is being produced because of a minor hormonal irregularity which will correct itself in time. This can be overcome by the use of a cream called KY jelly. It can be bought from any chemist without a prescription. This lubricant jelly should be smeared round the inside of the entrance to the vagina and round the labia prior to intercourse, and as it is water soluble and entirely harmless, it can be particularly helpful for your kind of problem.